# EXERCISES
## FOR
# PARKINSON'S
# DISEASE

# EXERCISES
## FOR
# PARKINSON'S DISEASE

### The Complete Fitness Guide to Improve Mobility and Wellness

WILLIAM SMITH, M.S.

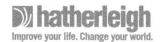

Improve your life. Change your world.

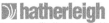
Improve your life. Change your world.

Hatherleigh Press is committed to preserving and protecting
the natural resources of the earth. Environmentally responsible and
sustainable practices are embraced within the company's
mission statement.

Visit us at www.hatherleighpress.com and register online for free
offers, discounts, special events, and more.

Library of Congress Cataloging-in-Publication Data is available upon request.
ISBN: 978-1-57826-766-8

*Interior Design by Cynthia Dunne*

Printed in the United States
20  19  18  17  16  15  14  13  12  11

getfitnow

Your health starts here! Workouts, nutrition, motivation,
community . . . everything you need to build a better body
from the inside out!

Visit us at www.getfitnow.com for videos, workouts, nutrition, recipes,
community tips, and more!

Consult your physician before beginning any exercise program. The author and publisher of this book and workout disclaim any liability, personal or professional, resulting from the misapplication of any of the following procedures described in this publication.

# CONTENTS

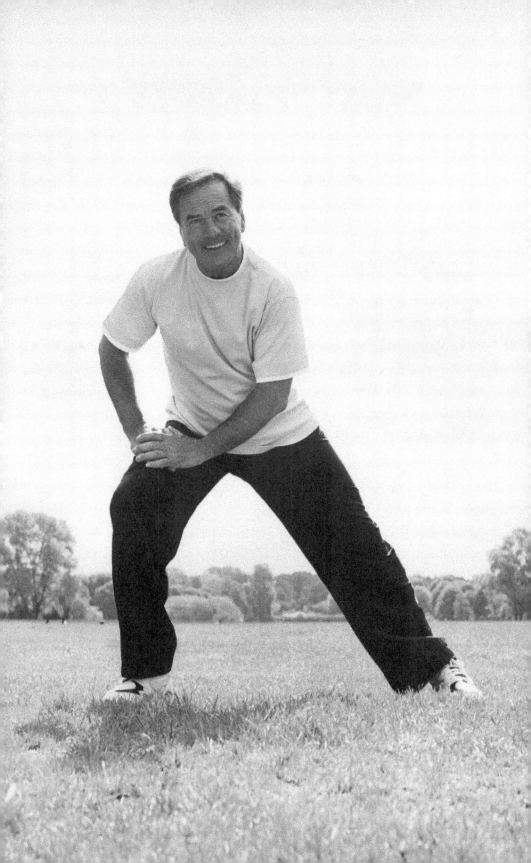

# CHAPTER 1

# Understanding Parkinson's Disease

Approximately 60,000 people are diagnosed with Parkinson's disease (PD) in the United States annually. However, while a diagnosis of Parkinson's will certainly bring about changes in a person's lifestyle, it is very possible to live a long and healthy life in spite of the disease. But to do so, patients, their family members, and healthcare providers must develop a proactive plan to manage the progression of the disease and help maintain the person's high quality of life for many years to come.

This plan should include healthy lifestyle choices and aim for far-reaching beneficial effects. Of course, it is important for people from all walks of life to develop good habits, such as maintaining a nutritious diet and remaining physically active. However, it is especially important for people living with PD to make those healthy choices that will enable them to better manage their symptoms and side effects in the long term. While medication can be used to lessen the early effects of Parkinson's, exercise can help combat long-term ailments like muscle rigidity, balance deterioration, and fatigue, which are often associated with the disease as it progresses.

For these and other benefits, it is important that patients with PD start an exercise program early on as part of a complete approach to treating their illness. In this chapter, you will find information about common symptoms and side effects that present in individuals living with Parkinson's disease. In addition to descriptions of these symptoms, you will find practical tips for managing their effects and improving your quality of life.

## DEFINING PARKINSON'S DISEASE

Parkinson's disease is a neurodegenerative disorder that impacts certain key nerve cells in the human brain. Normally, these cells produce dopamine, a chemical that sends signals to the part of the brain that controls movement. PD causes these dopamine-producing nerve cells to break down, which leads to difficulty in controlling movement. While experts are still unsure of what exactly causes the loss of these neurons, current research is focused on studying genetic markers and environmental factors.

Symptoms of PD generally appear in people between the ages of 50–65 years old, but they can sometimes appear earlier. Early symptoms of Parkinson's are diagnosed in stages, and can be so subtle and varied that the disease may go unnoticed for years. Since it takes time to develop the more obvious motor symptoms, such as hand tremors, early detection is essential to confirm the correct diagnosis and initiate treatment. When there is a family history of the disease, it is important to inform one's health professionals so they can look for any possible early indicators. These symptoms tend to begin on one side of the body and progress slowly, usually over a number of years. Parkinson's is both a chronic and progressive disease, meaning it persists over a long period and symptoms become more pronounced over time. Research has also shown that Parkinson's can impact non-dopamine producing cells in the brain, which contributes to some of the non-movement symptoms and side effects that may emerge.

> **THE FIVE STAGES OF PARKINSON'S DISEASE**
>
> **Stage One:** Mild symptoms, such as tremors or limb shaking. Poor posture, loss of balance, and unusual facial expressions.
>
> **Stage Two:** The symptoms become bilateral, affecting both limbs and both sides of the body. Problems emerge with walking and/or balance and completing regular tasks.
>
> **Stage Three:** Stage Three symptoms become more difficult to manage as they include the inability to walk straight or even stand. Movement becomes strained and slow.
>
> **Stage Four:** This stage is marked by a severely limited ability to walk as rigidity and bradykinesia (a slowing of movement) often prevail. Most patients are rendered unable to complete tasks, and typically cannot live independently. The tremors or shakiness of the earlier stages of the disease may lessen or even go away all together for unknown reasons.
>
> **Stage Five:** A person at Stage Five (and occasionally Stage Four) requires one-on-one caregivers, if not nursing care, and guidance from medical professionals.

In the next section, you will find some common symptoms and side effects of PD, along with practical suggestions for improving one's health designed specifically for those living with it. It is important to note that PD does not affect everyone the same way, and that symptoms, signs, and severity will vary from person to person.

## MOTOR SYMPTOMS

### Tremors

Tremors, or shaking, is one of the most common early symptoms of Parkinson's and is reported by about 80 percent of people with the disease. Tremors frequently begin in the upper body, usually in the hand or fingers, though sometimes a foot or the jaw may be affected first. Many people will often experience what is called a "pill-rolling" tremor, which is a back-and-forth rubbing of the thumb and index finger.

In the early stages of Parkinson's, tremors will usually appear on one side of the body; as the disease progresses, they will begin to appear on both sides. Tremors are most commonly observed when the limb is at rest or when a person is experiencing increased stress levels. Usually, tremors will disappear with deliberate movement, which means this symptom is not necessarily limiting in terms of functionality for people with PD.

**Tips for managing tremors:**

- Stabilize your arms on a flat surface whenever possible. For example, when combing your hair or eating, place your elbows on the table. Doing so will also help prevent upper body fatigue.
- Sit down to complete everyday tasks such as brushing your teeth or cooking. Not only does sitting help reduce the risk of falling, it also enables the body to better manage upper body tremors.
- Work on managing stress, frustration, and anxiety, which often exacerbate tremors associated with PD. When you are feeling particularly stressed, try deep breathing exercises and relaxation techniques to allow the nervous system to reset, which may help lessen tremors. Try the two breathing techniques detailed in the box below and remember to take your time when completing everyday tasks, as rushing will only increase stress and frustration.
- Keep a record or journal, noting the time of day when your tremors are mild and when they are severe. Try to plan your daily activities around those times when your tremors seem to be at their weakest.
- Finally, keep busy; most tremors will subside with intentional movement. Try squeezing a stress ball in the affected hand to manage a tremor.

### TRY IT NOW: BREATHING EXERCISES

Early onset PD often affects the neck and shoulder muscles, which can result in shallow breathing. As PD progresses and symptoms spread throughout the body, posture instability sometimes impedes the diaphragm and complicates breathing functions in the midsection of the body. Both simple and deep breathing exercises are important for people in the early and late stages of the disease. Try these breathing exercises, which have a calming effect and can help with muscle tension and rigidity.

Here's a simple breathing exercise: Take a slow, deep breath in through your nose, and then exhale slowly through your mouth. Despite the simplicity of this breathing exercise, this technique will help slow your heart rate, relax your body, and calm your mind. Often, people grow accustomed to short, shallow breathing throughout the course of their day. Deep breathing is much more effective for the body and will lead to increased relaxation.

Now for a deep breathing exercise: Close your eyes and take normal, deep breaths in through your nose. Concentrate on filling your lower abdomen with air. It may be helpful to place a hand on the lower abdomen to help you focus on breathing deeply and filling it. Hold that air in for 5–7 seconds. Then, in a controlled, slow manner, exhale out of your mouth as silently as possible. Try this practice for approximately five minutes every day to help relax your body and calm your mind.

## ALTERNATE NOSTRIL BREATHING

Requiring a bit more effort to learn, the practice of **alternate nostril breathing** can not only enhance overall health and well-being, but can also have a positive impact on your physical and physiological health by improving neurocognitive, respiratory, metabolic and nervous system functions in healthy people.

To practice alternate nostril breathing, sit comfortably with your legs crossed in the pretzel position, if possible. Place your left hand on your left knee and lift your right hand toward your nose. Exhale completely, then close your right nostril with your right thumb.

Now inhale through your left nostril and then close the left nostril with your fingers. Open the right nostril and exhale through this side. Inhale through the right nostril and then close this nostril. Open the left nostril and exhale through the left side.

This constitutes one cycle. Continue for up to 5 minutes, always completing the practice by finishing with an exhale from the left nostril.

## Slowness of Movement (Bradykinesia)

Bradykinesia refers to a slowness of movement and an impaired ability to move quickly on command, and is commonly associated with PD. This symptom often develops early in the disease but is usually subtle, at least in the initial stages. Bradykinesia can present as a reduced arm swing, shorter steps while walking, hesitation when initiating movement, smaller handwriting, or a reduced blink rate. This symptom of PD can make simple, everyday tasks such as getting up out of a chair or buttoning a shirt more complicated. Bradykinesia may also lead to a lack of animated facial expressions, which can often be misinterpreted by others as disinterest in what they are doing or saying.

**Tips for managing Bradykinesia:**

- Engage in regular aerobic exercises such as walking or swimming to help build your strength and balance.
- Focus on flexibility by regularly stretching, yoga, Tai chi, and foam rolling starting with a soft roller.
- Eat a healthy, balanced diet is recommended. Nutritional considerations include emphasizing plant-based proteins, minimizing animal fat, and staying hydrated.
- Oxidative stress can result from inflammation caused by stress, nutrition or environmental factors. Manage inflammation with a wide array of foods that include lentils, broccoli, spinach, blueberries and cherries.

## Rigid Muscles

Rigidity, or resistance to movement, is another recurring symptom that people with Parkinson's disease often report. Muscle stiffness can occur on one or both sides of the body, as well as in any part of the body. This symptom limits a person's range of motion. Often, a person feels tightness in the limbs and may experience aches or pain in the affected muscles or joints. Rigidity is a symptom that often directly impacts a person's quality of life, but there are simple steps you can take to lessen its severity.

### Tips for managing rigidity:

- Stay active throughout the day. Movement will improve motor symptoms, which helps prevent stiff muscles.
- Incorporate a flexibility component into your daily exercise routine. Consider Tai chi or yoga to help you stretch your trunk and limbs while increasing your range of motion.
- Try using heat to relax muscles. A warm bath or heating pad may help loosen up tensed muscles.
- Consider getting a massage. Massages may help manage pain and stress.

## Postural Instability

People in the later stages of Parkinson's often experience impaired balance and stooped posture. A person with postural instability will have trouble with balance, walking, and turning around. Some may develop a tendency to sway backward when rising from a chair or experience "freezing," where it feels as if their feet are glued to the floor. It is important to discuss postural instability with a doctor because it can lead to an increased risk of falling and fall-related injuries, such as broken bones. Postural instability symptoms do not always respond well to anti-Parkinson's medications, but may be helped by exercises specifically designed to improve balance.

**Tips for managing postural instability:**

- Consider an adaptive aid, such as a cane, which can help you improve your posture and balance while walking.
- Participate in stretching the front chest and neck muscles to promote a more upright posture.
- Try light strength training exercises to help strengthen back muscles and keep you in a more upright posture.
- Perform Calf/Shin Raise (Double Leg or Single Leg). Position your heels so that they are hanging off the stairs. Gently lift the heels up and slowly down. These muscles help in walking and balance.

## Core Instability

Core stability and posture go hand and hand. Thus, postural instability is undoubtedly linked to inactive trunks or "core muscles," and muscles that do not function properly during movements such as walking, stair climbing and getting up/down from sitting positions. Parkinson's patients present with a variety of mobility changes linked to postural instability. These challenges may include, but are not limited to: a shuffling gait, forward trunk lean, shortened arm swing and an inability to make concise directional changes.

The core has traditionally been thought of as the muscles in the stomach located between the ribs and pelvis, hence the propensity for crunches and sit-ups. We now know that "core strength" is a complex inner-working of joints, muscles, and connective tissue, all controlled by the nervous system.

So, for PD, we have to think globally, from the feet to the head. The "core" is a conduit between the upper and lower extremities, and how they provide balance during static and dynamic movements is crucial. As a point of reference, think of the core as being located between the shoulders and knees, yet responsive in activating all movement from the feet to the head. This may seem a bit complex; it may help to think of muscles as students, and the nervous system as the teacher. Hence, muscles only do what the central nervous system (brain and spinal cord) tells them to do. Thus, in the case of PD, exercises that integrate into improvements in whole body function are ideal.

It's generally agreed in the field of movement science that well-coordinated core muscles stabilize the spine and help create a firm base of support for healthy, effective movement. Stimulating the body with new activities, whether mental or physical, is vital to healthy development. Core training has become part of a larger method of training commonly referred to as functional training.

**Functional training** uses dynamic movements that involve lunging, pressing, pushing, pulling, extension, squatting, and rotating. These movements use a combination of stability (maintained position) and mobility (movement through space) to achieve a given task. For example, consider the actions involved in starting a lawn mower. You start with a wide stance, tighten your core, and pull the handle-cord, which starts the motor. This motion is an example of combining stability and mobility.

We perform hundreds of these movements every day—some subtle, others more complicated and challenging.

**Tips for maintaining balance include:**

- Try to keep one hand free at all times. Use a backpack or fanny pack to hold important items rather than carrying them in both hands as you move from room to room.
- Use both of your arms, swinging them if possible, to balance your gait. And try to lift your feet off of the ground when walking to avoid shuffling or dragging your feet which can throw you off balance.
- When standing, keep your feet shoulder width apart to maintain a steady posture. Don't wear rubber soled shoes as they may stick to the floor and cause trips.
- Count to 15 seconds between movements such as standing from a seated position before you begin walking. If it's all too hard, consider using a walking aid until you are ready to try again.

## NON-MOTOR SYMPTOMS

### Urinary Problems or Constipation

Chronic constipation and urinary problems are commonly caused by PD. Many people will experience constipation, a condition where a person is unable to empty their bowels due to the improper functioning of the autonomic nervous system, which regulates smooth muscle control. People may also experience difficulty controlling their bladder or have trouble urinating. Constipation and urinary problems can cause pain and discomfort, but there are things you can do to lessen the severity of these side effects.

**Tips for managing urinary problems or constipation:**

- Changes in diet may help alleviate constipation. Increasing your fiber intake makes it easier for waste to pass through the intestines. Talk to your doctor about making nutritional changes that will work for you.
- Increasing your water or sparkling water intake will also help ease constipation. Avoid caffeinated beverages like soda or coffee, which may worsen urinary problems. If getting up at night to use the bathroom is a problem, consider limiting fluid intake two hours before bedtime.
- Engage in light exercise, like going for regular walks, to help stimulate slowed bowels.
- Talk to your doctor about the medications you are taking. Sometimes constipation can be a side effect of prescription medications.

### Fatigue

Many people with PD experience loss of energy and fatigue. Fatigue is a feeling of weariness and lethargy that persists over a long period of time and is not alleviated simply by rest. Fatigue can impact your physical, mental, and emotional well-being. People living with Parkinson's often experience fatigue that is made worse by muscle rigidity, slow and labored movement, depression, and sleep disorders, which are all common side effects of PD.

**Tips for managing fatigue:**

- Eat a healthy, balanced diet to help you feel energized.
- Participate in light aerobic exercise to help increase energy, being careful not to overload yourself.
- A short nap at midday can be helpful and refreshing, but try not to sleep too long or take too many naps, as that may make sleeping at night more difficult.

- Participate in mentally stimulating activities, like doing a crossword puzzle, to help stave off boredom, which often contributes to feelings of fatigue.
- Keep track of when your energy levels are high and when they are waning. Plan your day around your body's tendencies so that you can get important activities done when you are at your peak.
- Spend time outside, taking in the sunlight and fresh air. This will help invigorate your senses and lift your energy and mood.
- Know your limitations and don't be ashamed to ask for help when you need it.

## Sleep Deprivation

Sleep is becoming an endangered resource in our society. We live busier and busier lives that motivate us to work harder and longer. Sleep deprivation has been linked to an increased risk of cardiovascular diseases, slower reflexes, and negative mental functioning in the brain.

The National Institute of Health (NIH) estimates 60 million Americans have insomnia frequently or for extended periods of time. The NIH also indicates sleep problems affect virtually every aspect of day-to-day living including mood, mental alertness, work performance, and energy level.

Sleep deprivation has direct links to impairments in concentration, memory, and cognitive function. Sleep acts as medicine for the brain, healing brain tissue that is under constant stress, both good and bad. Think of the brain as a computer that must shut down and "reboot." This allows for the down time the body needs for rest, recovery, and stimulating the five stages of sleeping cycles (culminating in REM and NREM sleep).

Research recommends we get between 7–8 hours of sleep every night. We know that sleep and memory are intimately linked, but what if someone is not getting their daily dose? Drugs, herbal remedies, and sleep clinics are often recommended.

**Simple steps to promote quality sleep include the following:**

- Avoid stimulants such as caffeine, alcohol, and chocolates before bed.
- Schedule more vigorous workouts earlier in the day.

As with Parkinson's, repetition in activities is very important. Try to go to bed every night at the same time, take naps at regular intervals, and avoid sleeping during the day unless it feels unavoidable.

## Cognitive Changes

Although Parkinson's primarily affects dopamine generation in the brain, non-dopamine producing brain cells can be impacted as well. As a result, cognitive changes may occur in individuals diagnosed with PD even before motor symptoms become obvious. These changes may appear as problems maintaining attention, planning, problem-solving, speaking, or issues with memory. Thankfully, there are adaptive strategies you can implement in your daily life to lessen the impact of these changes.

**Tips for managing cognitive changes:**

- Make "to-do" lists and notes in a calendar or planner to help you remember important dates, appointments, and other essential information.
- Keep important items, such as your keys or glasses, in the same location to help avoid the frustration of misplacing them.
- Stay cognitively active by exercising your brain. Attempt a crossword puzzle, read a book, or play a card game to stimulate your brain.
- Stay social and make time to interact with people on a regular basis. Call friends or family, join a group exercise class, or visit the local library.
- Use alarms or timers to help you remember your medication schedule.

**TRY IT NOW: FUN ACTIVITIES**

With so many options to support daily cognitive health, here is one thing that you can do right now, even if you're not currently doing anything else. Pick one activity that you enjoy, and make this activity a daily habit.

The underlying premise here is consistency. By performing this activity on a daily basis, it will become a habit in around 25 days. The consistency accomplishes a second task: **motor learning**. By executing a task with consistency, you can develop a new motor pattern, refine a current motor pattern or take the opportunity to correct old, unhealthy patterns. An example pertaining specifically to Parkinson's is directional change. Walk forward, stop, pivot left or right, then walk again for a few steps. This drill integrates stride, body awareness, change of direction, and uses the upper/lower body together.

## Mood Disorders: Depression and Anxiety

It is not uncommon for people with PD to experience emotional and psychological side effects, which often manifest themselves in the form of mood disorders. The two most commonly reported mood disorders are depression and anxiety.

Parkinson's disease and depression often coexist. Depression may result from the social isolation that can occur when chronic physical conditions contribute to a loss of physical independence, resulting in a significant impact upon one's mental and physical health. Depression should be considered alongside smoking and obesity as a major risk factor to health. The combination of social, physical, and cognitive stressors should be monitored as contributors to high levels of stress, which in the long term can result in inflammatory response, an underlying contributor to many chronic diseases, including Parkinson's.

Depression goes well beyond mere sadness and is often characterized by severe feelings of worthlessness, guilt, or hopelessness that persist over an extended period of time. Depression, in the case of Parkinson's patients, often goes underdiagnosed and undertreated, so it is important to keep the lines of communication open with your doctor. The mental and emotional experience of having Parkinson's is the hardest to wrap one's mind around. For this reason, it is the role of a psychologist to help you sort out the layers of depression that clog up your mental and behavioral health, and provide therapy to deal with anxiety and stress. As many as 40 percent of people living with Parkinson's will experience depression at some point as their disease progresses.

Anxiety is a common emotion that many people experience at different points in their lives. However, when feelings of mild to severe fear, dread, and nervousness consistently interfere with your normal life, it is important to acknowledge and address it with a doctor.

### Tips for managing mood disorders:

- Limit alcohol and caffeine intake, opting for water instead.
- Eat well-balanced meals and healthy snacks.
- Staying well-rested is important. You should aim for 8 hours of sleep per night.
- Exercise can help boost your mood and keep you energized and healthy.
- Try deep breathing and relaxation exercises when you are feeling particularly irritable or stressed to help relieve tension and refocus yourself.
- Talk to someone about what you are feeling or experiencing. It is okay to ask for help. In some cases, your doctor may be able prescribe medication to help treat depression and anxiety.

Controlling risk factors, including stress, allows the body to fully realize the full benefits of regular physical activities. Time and time again, "mind-body" connection exercises have been shown to enhance mental acuity, focus, and brain function.

### Sleep Disorders

Getting adequate sleep is essential to a person's physical, mental, and emotional well-being. Sadly, people who are living with PD often have to cope with any number of sleep disruptions. They may struggle to fall asleep at night or have difficulty staying asleep, making it a challenge to get a good night's rest. Combinations of other Parkinson's side effects can also make it difficult to sleep.

Sleep is when your brain recharges from the day's events and new neural pathways develop. Considering that Parkinson's is a neurodegenerative disease, allowing your central nervous system the time it needs to rest and recover is critical. Poor sleeping habits have been linked to a variety of co-morbidities and risk factors not directly related to Parkinson's, such as elevated cortisol levels, general lethargy and low-grade fatigue, decreased mental acuity, and changes in muscle tone/body composition.

**Tips for managing sleep disorders:**

- Create a consistent sleep routine by going to bed at the same time and waking up around the same time each day. Aim for 7–8 hours of sleep, but do not sleep much longer than 8 hours.
- Train your brain and body to associate your bed with sleep. Do not lie in bed to watch television or read.
- Avoid drinking liquids two hours before bed and try to use the restroom right before you retire for the night.
- Avoid drinking caffeinated beverages like soda or coffee, especially in the evenings.
- Try simple breathing exercises before bed to help you relax and fall asleep more easily.
- Avoid technology, like cell phones or tablets, right before bed. The light emitted from these devices suppresses the production of melatonin, a hormone that controls your sleep and wake cycles.
- Include light to moderate exercise in your day but avoid heavy physical activity 1–2 hours prior to going to sleep.
- Spend time outside in the sunshine. Fresh air and sunlight will help keep your internal clock on the right track.

The first step to creating a comprehensive lifestyle plan to help mitigate symptoms of Parkinson's and strengthen your body is to have a more complete understanding of the illness and its side effects. The next step, which we'll explore in the following chapter, is to find those lifestyle habits which you can cultivate and stick to, and which work best for you and your specific health care needs.

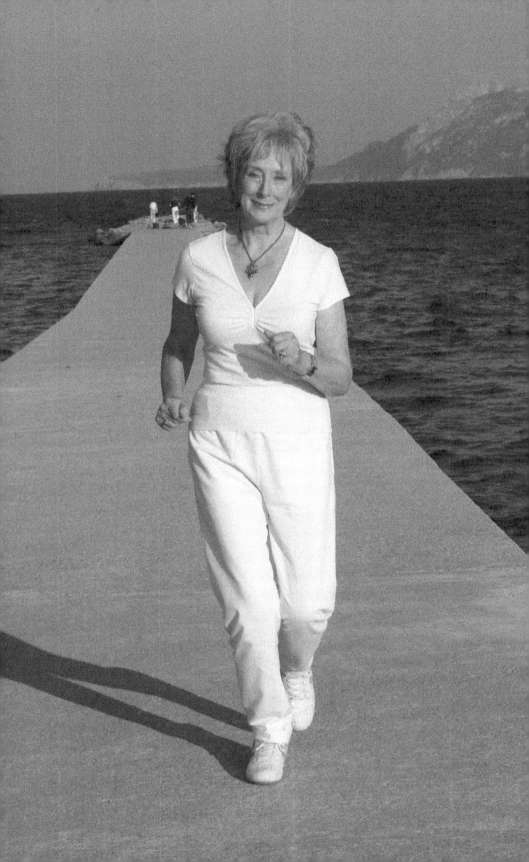

# CHAPTER 2

# Maintaining a Healthy Brain

We often overlook the importance of lifestyle (for example, nutrition and exercise) when it comes to brain health. In this chapter, we will discuss some of the many lifestyle, environmental, and genetic factors that can impact one's likelihood of developing Parkinson's and how you can help your loved ones to control their preventable risk factors, in order to obtain a better quality of life.

For example: we often associate the stress response in the body to work or family activities that place us in situations that are unpleasant. But the stress response, also known as 'fight-or-flight,' can also be caused by poor nutritional intake. Sub-optimal nutritional intake leads to increased acidity in the blood, chemical and hormonal imbalances, and ultimately an acidic environment that destroys neurons in the brain.

The question then becomes: How do we create a nurturing, nutrient-rich environment that fosters healthy brain tissue?

## CALORIE RESTRICTION

Seventy years ago, research suggested that **calorie restriction** is linked to the prevention of various chronic diseases, including heart disease, Parkinson's, and Alzheimer's disease. These conditions are generally age-related, not age-dependent; in other words, it should not be assumed that these ailments afflict an individual simply because they have reached a certain age. Parkinson's, for example, commonly affects geriatric populations but is not a normal part of aging. Recent research has reinforced the link between reducing caloric intake and disease prevention. This, combined with recent advancements in medical treatment and an enhanced understanding of how these illnesses affect the body, means we have a unique opportunity to prevent certain dementia-like diseases. This means that reducing caloric intake is key to taking an active role in preventing these diseases.

The connection between calorie restriction and disease prevention has been studied for over 50 years, and the evidence remains relevant today. Scientists have discovered that when animals are forced to live on 30–40 percent fewer calories than they would normally consume, they become resistant to most age-related diseases and live 30–50 percent longer. It's easy to see how this research is potentially relevant to humans. While research results in mice do not always prove true in humans, this is often the case.

## HYDRATION: WATER INTAKE AND BRAIN HEALTH

Hydrate, hydrate, hydrate! 60 percent of our body mass is comprised of water, and our brain is 80 percent water in content. As Parkinson's is a disease which encompasses the brain, spinal cord, and nerves, **hydration** is an essential step to prevent the development of the disease. Every other important piece of the human body relies heavily on water, or the fluids it makes up such as cerebrospinal fluid (CSP). Our brains sit in CSP, which bathes, lubricates, and hydrates the convoluted folds of the brain itself.

Maintaining proper hydration levels is one approach to disease prevention that is within our control. That means we should take in half of our body weight, or 25–30 percent, through our diet. This is equivalent to 6–8 8-ounce glasses of water per day. Having water on hand while traveling or during physical activity, for example, is one easy way to increase the likeliness of fluid intake. This is particularly important for those with Parkinson's, who may not reach the same activity levels of those without the condition, thereby decreasing their fluid intake below what is needed to maintain healthy brain function.

With that said, you should drink often, even when you're not thirsty. By the time you experience thirst, your body has already been deprived of the hydration it needs for some time. Remember, don't let your loved one wait until they're parched to drink water; instead, encourage them to drink water before dehydration symptoms occurs.

In addition, keep tabs on visible feedback of hydration, including urine color, skin pliability, and normal sweating. Urine color should be pale to light in color, while skin pliability should stretch and return to normal texture immediately. Sweating can be an additional indication of proper hydration. Sweating during exercise and physical activity is normal and expected. Exercise without sweating, while possible, is not a regular occurrence.

## MANAGING STRESS THROUGH MEDITATION

Focusing on the breath is one of the most common and fundamental techniques for accessing a meditative state, one which helps us to mitigate the ill effects of stress and gather our energy to overcome daily challenges. Breathing is part of a deep rhythm of the body that connects us intimately with the world around us. Learn these steps, and then share them with someone you care for.

Close your eyes, breathe deeply and regularly, and observe your breath as it flows in through the nose and out of the mouth. Give your full attention to the breath as it comes in, and full attention to the breath as it goes out. Store your breath in the belly, not the chest, between inhales and exhales. Whenever you find your attention wandering away from your breath, gently pull it back to the rising and falling of the breath in the belly.

Inhale through your nose slowly and deeply, feeling the lower chest and abdomen inflate like a balloon. Hold for 5 seconds. Exhale deeply, deflating the lower chest and abdomen like in emptying balloon. Hold for 5 seconds. Do this five times, and then allow your breathing to return to a normal rhythm.

You will begin to feel a change come over your entire body. Gradually, you will become less aware of your breathing, but not captured in your stream of consciousness. Often we are too alert and hyper-stimulated by TV, caffeine, and family life, just to name a few causes. By breathing mindfully for 5 minutes daily, you will become more centered inward. You will live "in the moment," in your own skin.

**Benefits of simple breathing exercises throughout the day include:**

- Calming
- "Re-centering" one's thoughts
- Increase in oxygenated blood flow, improved efficiency expiring carbon dioxide
- Decreased levels of fatigue later in the day, legs won't feel "heavy"

Increasing oxygenated blood via deep breathing can decrease muscle pains, especially in the postural muscles (back and neck muscles), and help counteract chronic stressors such as sitting or standing and static positions for extended periods of time.

## DECREASING INFLAMMATION: FREE RADICALS, ANTIOXIDANTS, AND AGING CELLS

Many of us have heard the term **inflammation**, but what exactly is it? The body's pH is the measurement of alkalinity or acidity in the body's biochemistry—specifically the fluid environment, such as blood or spinal fluid, that exists throughout the body. The key is to find a balance in the body between the necessary acidity found in the stomach, for example, while keeping low acidity in the intestine and blood.

**Factors that contribute to inflammation:**

- Stress, both good (eustress) and bad (distress)
- Inadequate or erratic sleep patterns
- Poor nutrition from trans/saturated fats, processed foods, refined carbohydrates
- Diuretics, i.e. drinking excess soda, tea/coffee, water pills
- Food supply chain, from genetically modified foods, hormone injected animals/foods

- Environment, such as living in urban areas, smog-centric geography
- Medications

Following a high fiber, lean protein, whole grain, and anti-inflammatory diet is key to brain health. The Integrative Medicine Program at the Atlantic Health System in New Jersey provides very specific guidelines to apply to day-to-day healthy brain nutritional intake. In particular, they advise avoiding high-fructose corn syrup and simple or additive sugared foods as much as possible. Sugar is poison to brain and blood, as exemplified by the connection between diabetes and dementia.

Sugar has no purpose other than to change and enhance taste. Find another way to achieve the same purpose by replacing sugar with agave or honey. Also look out for carbohydrates, typically white in color, that turn to sugar in the body. These can include noodles, certain breads, and rice. The body has to expend (waste) precious energy to process these foods. A few common foods to avoid would be candy, some cereals, ice cream, jam/ jelly, doughnuts, and pie.

**Additional strategies to stabilize pH and decrease long-term inflammatory diseases (such as cancer) include:**

- Consume a variety of colorful fruits and vegetables (favoring dark, leafy vegetables)
- Drink 6–8 glasses of fluid (water, natural juices, dark teas).
- Favor non-red meat sources, including fish.
- Consume good fats, including Omega 3's, 6's, deep-water fatty fishes, flax seeds, and tree nuts, like walnuts, Brazil nuts, pecans, and pistachios.
- Eat blueberries, blackberries, goji berries, cranberries, and elderberries for their antioxidant qualities.
- Do not overcook foods; this de-natures, or breaks down, the protein bond and makes the food source more unstable before it enters the body.
- Increase consumption of antioxidants, which work to deter the impact of oxidants that contribute to cellular aging (i.e. aging, brain death, and basically getting old).

## FRUITS, VEGETABLES, AND COLORFUL FOODS

**Natural foods,** which basically means anything which is unprocessed, comes from the ground, and raised organically, are great. That said, organic foods are not the only way to go; but if there is an option between foods raised with pesticides or genetically modified foods, it's in your loved one's best interest to pursue the least chemically-laced product.

A balanced diet is important in providing your body with the fuel for maintaining the strength necessary to deal with Parkinson's. The stronger the body, the easier it will be. Keeping a nutrition journal for a week is one excellent approach to evaluating your diet. A simple chart of your food intake over a week will give you a better idea of what it takes for a balanced diet.

As a start, fiber, antioxidants, and phytochemicals are in plentiful supply in dark leafy vegetables, red peppers, spaghetti squash, bean varieties, and electrolyte-rich bananas. Bananas are also high in B vitamins that support the nervous system.

## BUILDING A BETTER BRAIN

**Brain health** in relation to aging is a hot-button topic. The Population Reference Bureau indicates that 1 in 12 elderly people experience a decline in cognitive function so severe they have difficulty performing the normal activities of daily living, and eventually, cannot live independently.

Forgetting where you placed your keys or questioning whether you turned off the lights are common, everyday concerns for people of all ages. Yet in the case of key portions of the aging population, this occasional absent-mindedness translates to an observable decline in their cognitive ability, as they suddenly forget their own phone number, or can't recall how to get home from the job they've worked at for 20 years.

Thankfully, the decline of brain health doesn't have to be a normal part of aging. Researcher Kenneth Langa at the University of Michigan School of Medicine and Institute for Social Research has found that education levels seem to be a determinant in cognitive health as we age. Langa concluded that individuals with higher levels of education are at a lesser risk of suffering cognitive decline.

What this means is that by keeping your brain sharp by continuing to learn—no matter your education level—is always important to preventing the onset of brain related diseases. Continuing to learn and building a "buff brain" is possible, and should be part of any effort towards healthy living. New studies, which focus around fancy names like 'neuroplasticity' and 'neurogenesis,' are examining how the brain deforms and learns based on new stimuli by creating new connections between neurons.

And the best part is that much of this positive research on brain health is pointing to exercise as the key foundational element to support a healthier brain, as well as a healthier body. But before we get into the role of exercise in Parkinson's treatment, let's explore a few of the complementary therapies and environmental factors that can help tie everything together to create that comprehensive lifestyle plan we're looking for.

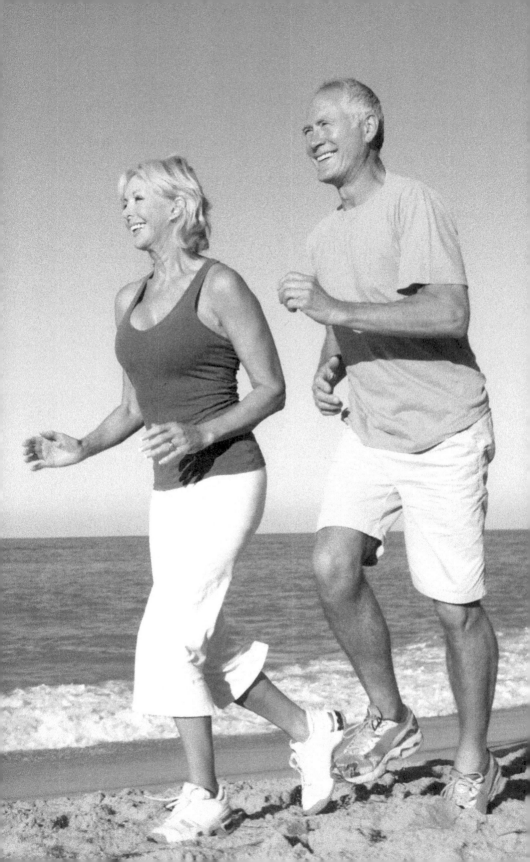

# CHAPTER 3

---

# Therapy
# and Support

Parkinson's disease is a progressive condition, and the responsibility of caring for a loved one can often last for many years. This takes its toll on the physical, emotional, and mental health of both the caregiver and the person afflicted. If you are currently caring for a loved one with dementia and feel a need to establish a greater support system, don't wait. Friends, family members, community members, and church organizations are just a few examples of resources to explore.

## DEVELOPING SOCIAL SUPPORT SYSTEMS

**Companionship** and **a connectedness with one's surroundings** is vital to those with Parkinson's. Having a support system (for example, a dependable neighbor or a family member) in place so that a patient can receive assistance in activities (such as the administration of daily medications or performing daily exercises) is especially important in enhancing the quality of life for those with the disease.

Similarly, healthy living is important for both the caregiver and the afflicted person. This includes reaching out to others for additional support when needed, staying organized with to-do lists, and paying close attention to your own stress levels.

Getting out of the house and meeting people should be the first step. Opening up the world of a person stricken with Parkinson's by meeting other people will completely change their outlook on life. We know that isolation from others can lead to depression, which compounds symptoms. Those endorphins (a.k.a. the body's natural pain medication) are released through fulfilling, happy experiences. By engaging friendly and caring individuals, the patient reinforces the healthy neural connections and creates new ones.

Likewise, communicating feelings and emotions openly between the family and a person with Parkinson's is often difficult yet necessary. Listening can often be the most important skill a caregiver demonstrates. Nonverbal communication patterns from someone with dementia include abnormal lethargy, withdrawal from normally enjoyable activities, and forgetting names of loved ones are not only risk factors, but are also signs the disease is progressing.

Establishing a network of close relationships for Parkinson's patients is an excellent strategy that will support the physical and mental exercises contained in this book's program.

## TIPS FOR CAREGIVERS

For caregivers, helping your patient or loved one get their day back on track can be as simple as following these 10 tips, intended to help smooth out the ups and downs in their daily schedule:

1. **Stretch** for 5 minutes before getting out of bed in the morning to prepare your muscles for movement.
2. **Lay your clothes out for the next day prior to going to bed.** Confusion is common first thing in the morning as the optic nerve and ocular muscles around the eyes have been in a state of relaxation throughout the night, so chances are that choosing matching clothes will not be an easy task to perform in the morning.

3. **Drink one large glass of water in the morning to stabilize your morning eating habits.** Our bodies are approximately 60 percent water. By replenishing the body first thing in the morning, the regulatory systems of our body, mainly heart rate and blood pressure, stay increasingly balanced.

4. **Eat 300–400 calories for breakfast.** Research has shown that eating breakfast improves memory performance.

5. **Stick to your diet, even when eating out.** Healthy lunch foods can easily be made to order at local restaurants. Pick steamed and broiled foods over fried. Gastrointestinal (GI) irritability can be exacerbated by fried and processed foods.

6. **Have an afternoon snack.** The afternoon is a perfect time to have a moderate carbohydrate/moderate protein-based snack or drink. An example would be a smoothie of dark berries with whey protein blended with water.

7. **Take a walk after dinner, remembering to wait 20–30 minutes after eating.** Stimulating blood flow through aerobically-based movement impact (not running) aids in the digestive process. Waiting 30 minutes allows the food to settle.

8. **Write a short to-do list before going to bed.** Keep your list to three priority items if you do not work and 1–2 priority items if you have a full-time occupation.

9. **Practice deep breathing as a form of relaxation before bed.** Deep breathing is an excellent way to slow the heart rate. Focus on breathing in through the nose and out through the mouth.

10. **Promote home safety.** The crucial concept here is setting up the home to minimize—or better still, totally remove—any risk of falling. Falling has a number of unhealthy consequences: injury, including broken bones, with the potential of being unable to exercise and all the attendant issues that raises, including life-threatening respiratory issues; and the emotional and mental toll over the loss of independence and fear of future falls.

## BUILD A NETWORK OF PROFESSIONAL CAREGIVERS

In addition to friends and family, professionals that have extensive experience and knowledge-based intellect in the field of Parkinson's are vital. This is hardly an all-inclusive list, so please refer to your primary care provider for additional information.

## Primary Care Physician

Primary care practitioners are coming back into vogue. The "medical home" model, in which the emphasis lies on a personal physician in a long-term medical relationship with the patient who is capable of acute, chronic and continuous and comprehensive care, is re-empowering the original provider of medical care. The trend over the last couple of decades has drifted away from the primary care doctor towards specialists that order expensive tests and scans. Having one point of contact is key to coordinating patient care.

## Neurologist

Neurologists are doctors that work with the nervous system and assessing its function. A neurologist is likely the medical provider that will provide the most clinical care to someone with Parkinson's disease.

## Psychologist or Psychiatrist

The mental aspects of Parkinson's are too extensive to list here. Given that the mental and physical aspects of the disease are substantial, having a mental health care professional on your support team is vital.

## Social Worker

Bringing a social worker in can help coordinate family and friends, along with the necessary medical care. Social workers become an integral part of the familial structure when there has been an injury or acute medical incident (stroke, fall, etc.) that has led to the one suffering with Parkinson's disease to become disabled.

## Physical and/or Occupational Therapist

Clinical rehabilitation (promoting a pain-free range of motion) and restoring function are the physical/occupational therapist's initial objectives. Their next goal is to establish an exercise program that can be used by the patient following treatment. Having their input can be invaluable when creating your comprehensive wellness plan.

## Fitness Professional

As a physical trainer, this category is dear to my heart! The personal trainer is the frontline of prevention. Listening, interpersonal communication skills, and knowledge-based skills are absolutes for quality personal trainers. Solid trainers have an excellent repertoire, and can work with both medical providers and colleagues in the fitness community.

## Adult Day Services Provider

Adult day services provide a variety of community-oriented services that emphasize the social experience overseen by complementary health and caregiver professionals. These day service centers provide socially uplifting activities during normal business hours. Many day services offer transportation, meals, snacks, personal care, and therapeutic activities.

## Home-Based Care Services

Similar to adult day services (in scope of practice), home-based care services may provide a cost-effective option to institutional care. Healthcare systems may offer this type of outreach program as an outpatient service or outsource to an outside contractor. Services may include 24-hour monitoring care, therapeutic services, daily activities and include grocery shopping, filling prescriptions, and cooking.

## Independent Living Facilities

These facilities have 24-hour services, medical response on-site (including nurses during scheduled times), and dining facilities. Private pay and subsidized care is generally available through state and federal government housing authorities.

## Assisted Living Residential Care

Assisted living care is the fastest growing segment of the geriatric/senior populations. Daily activities including bathing, washing, cooking, and dressing are provided for the resident. Closer, hands-on services are provided based on the level of disability or low level of functioning of the residents.

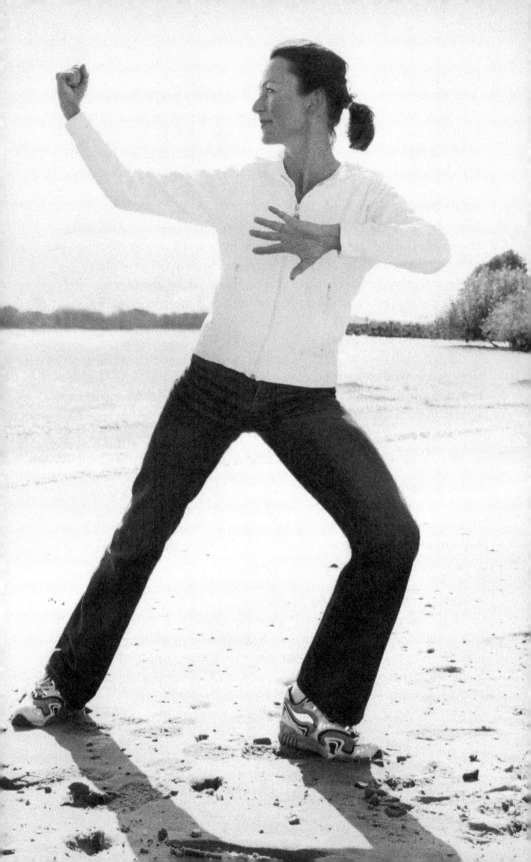

# CHAPTER 4

# Improving Wellness
# Through Exercise

Exercise is essential to maintaining overall health and wellness in all stages of life. Starting a regular exercise program can help prevent, delay, or manage a variety of health problems. The numerous benefits of exercise are well-documented: regular physical activity can boost your mood, strengthen your muscles and bones, and help improve brain function and memory.

For these reasons, it is especially important for someone with a chronic illness like Parkinson's disease to regularly engage in exercise and physical activity. While someone who struggles with symptoms of Parkinson's like fatigue and depression may not feel naturally inclined to engage in vigorous exercise, it is to your benefit to work with your doctor or physical therapist to find a workout program that is suited to your individual needs and goals. Even though exercise cannot cure Parkinson's, research has shown that exercise may be an effective strategy to delay the mobility decline that people living with the disease tend to experience.

## HOW DOES EXERCISE BENEFIT PEOPLE LIVING WITH PARKINSON'S DISEASE?

Starting an exercise routine can be both an effective and economical way to help combat some of the symptoms and side effects associated with Parkinson's disease. All people with Parkinson's, regardless of how far their illness has progressed, should consider beginning a workout routine.

Exercise can help improve balance, mobility, and strength, so that people with Parkinson's are better equipped to complete daily activities independently and have a higher quality of life. Additionally, the mental and emotional benefits of exercise can help boost mood and brain function.

**Other ways exercise benefits people with Parkinson's include:**

- Improvement of issues caused by the motor symptoms of PD
- Neuro-protective benefits; evidence suggests exercise may stimulate the production of nerve growth factors
- Stimulates the generation of stem cells in the brain and improves cognition
- Improves quality of sleep
- Increases endurance
- Increases awareness of proper body alignment and mechanics
- Improves breath support and control
- Builds healthy, strong bones
- Increases strength, especially in core stabilizing muscles like the abdominals and back
- Reduces fatigue and increases energy levels
- Affords a greater sense of well-being and improves self-esteem
- Improves ability to perform tasks
- Controls weight and burns calories

The earlier a Parkinson's patient can start a regular exercise program, the better. People often wait until they have mobility problems to begin exercising, but the sooner a person begins an exercise program designed to delay the onset of anticipated mobility problems, the more effective the program will be.

New research even suggests that people who have been diagnosed with Parkinson's can delay the onset of mobility impairment by adhering to an exercise program. Physical exercise improves disease symptoms, mobility, balance, gait, and overall quality of life, and a wide range of exercises, including tai-chi, boxing, dance, Pilates, kayaking, and agility training, can all have beneficial effects for people living with Parkinson's.

Medications manage the symptoms of Parkinson's but don't help the body produce dopamine on its own. Exercise is the best way to improve the quality of life and speech.

## WHAT TYPES OF EXERCISES BEST HELP PARKINSON'S SYMPTOMS?

The exercises outlined in Chapter 6 of this book have been carefully selected to improve mobility, increase flexibility, and strengthen muscles. Studies looking at aerobic exercise for potential neuroprotection have shown positive benefits as well for posture and rigidity.

These exercises target a range of Parkinson's symptoms, including (but not limited to): slowness of movement, tremors, stiffness, and postural instability.

Keep in mind that as you begin a new exercise program, it is important to start slowly and pace yourself. As you get more comfortable over time, you can begin to increase the intensity of your workouts. Always pay attention to how your body is responding to your exercise routine and only increase frequency and intensity when your body is ready for it. Pay attention to your symptoms, take breaks if you need to, but do not give up. You have so much to gain from your exercise program, including increased energy, improved balance and mobility, and a better quality of life.

**The following are some simple exercises to get you started:**

To Improve Mobility

> Quad Roller (page 90)
> Thoracic Flex (page 61)
> Overhead Squat (page 51)

To Increase Balance

> Foot Taps (page 92)
> Scissor Stretch (page 63)
> Heel to Toe Rocks (page 71)
> Stationary Lunge/Split Squat (page 81)

## To Improve Stability

Wall Sit with Foam Roller (page 54)
All 4s (page 94)
Deadbug (page 95)

## To Improve Flexibility

Scissor Stretch (page 63)
Hip Roller (page 89)
Cobra (page 85)
Double Arm Chest Stretch (page 76)

## To Improve Strength

Physioball Walk-Up (page 113)
Deadlift (page 56)
Lifting Movements with Band OR Push-ups (page 114 or 53)
Supermans (page 96)

## To Improve Reflexes

Heel to Toe Rocks (page 71)
Foot Taps (page 92)
Partner Stability Pushes: Sitting and Standing (page 77)
Single Arm Chest Press with Partner (page 76)

---

**PARKINSON'S FIT TIP: PARKINSON'S DISEASE DRILLS**
Practice these daily Parkinson's disease-specific "drills":
- Practice accentuated, long strides
- Practice navigating spaces with short strides
- Practice navigating stairs
- Practice shifting weight side-to-side, pausing momentarily

---

## POSTURE AND PARKINSON'S DISEASE

**Posture** is integral to all aspects of health, and sufferers of Parkinson's disease often struggle with maintaining a proper posture. The results of improper poster are wide-ranging, and include a number of persistent issues of muscle weakness, rigidity and lack of fine motor control, all of which are particularly concerning for a Parkinson's patient.

It's important to mention that everyone's spine is different, but the spine is generally the focal point when discussing posture. In respect to a healthy spine, you should have three anatomical curves: cervical, thoracic and lumbar. Parkinson's doesn't change the spine's anatomy— the three curves are still there in some form; rather, it changes how it performs its functions.

The **cervical spine** is comprised of seven vertebrae, beginning at the base of the skull and ending around where the neckline terminates into the shoulders. The "C-spine" rounds forward, allowing for dispersion of force placed upon the neck from the head. One cue is to look at the body from the side; your ear should be in line with your shoulder. This region of the spine is meant for mobility and stability. A common issue of the neck in people afflicted with Parkinson's is forward head posture. Long-term cervical misalignment may result in flattening curve or stress on the vertebrae from stenosis or arthritis.

The **thoracic spine** (or middle spine) has 12 vertebrae, beginning at the point where the C-spine stops. The T-spine is made for mobility, allowing for multiple other structures (ribs and shoulder blades) to attach and move. This region of the spine protects vital organs and acts as an intermediary between the lower and upper back. The middle spine is notorious for 'rounding forward' from excessive sitting, leading to poor posture. Parkinson's may cause musculoskeletal rigidity, with the resulting rounding and forward postural "lean" decreasing motor skill responsiveness. The altered posture in the mid-back may also lead to many long-term back discomfort.

The **lumbar spine** is comprised of five vertebrae, beginning in the lower back and ending where the back terminates into the pelvis (i.e. sacrum). These "L-spine" rounds are the largest of the vertebrae in the spine, which allow for the dispersion of compression force placed upon the back from both above and below. One cue when looking for these rounds is to look at the body from the side; you should see a natural curve forward. This region of the spine is meant for stability, supporting the body's load while also moving through all three planes of movement. The L-spine and pelvis are commonly referred to as the lumbo-pelvic girdle. Besides the close anatomical proximity, movement dysfunction can be traced to the hips and back. For example, lower back pain may begin in the hips or hip pain in the back.

## WHY POSTURAL IMPROVEMENTS MATTER FOR PARKINSON'S DISEASE

So, what are some of the benefits of engaging in a posture health improvement program?

Healthy posture—or a lack thereof—is one the first observational assessments health professionals make upon meeting a client. Determining whether a client has the ability to stand, sit and maintain upright positioning during movement provides valuable feedback on program design and recommendations for self-directed activity.

Environmental, lifestyle and possibly medical conditions may be cited as symptoms by clients with less than ideal postural alignment. For example, patients with poor posture may complain of difficulty breathing. It may be the case that their internal breathing mechanism is compressed due to their posture; this is particularly common in the case of kyphosis, or forward rounding. When forward rounding is present, it can make natural breathing quite difficult. Imagine a balloon that cannot fully inflate, placing tremendous pressure on one's internal anatomy.

When exerting your body, as during exercise, the physiological demands on the cardiovascular and respiratory systems become greater. When you cannot take deep breaths in or out during periods of physical exertion due to rounded posture, your ability to exhale carbon dioxide and inhale oxygen-rich air is diminished. This decreased function minimizes the body's ability to continue without frequent rest. Over time, this increased pressure raises blood pressure and resting heart rate.

The benefits of proper posture only become more significant as you age. Populations such as seniors, who have inherently diminished functional status due to aging, are put at greater risk of falls, vertigo and shortness of breath due to suboptimal postural alignment throughout their life.

Picture the ideal alignment as being the ear lined up over the shoulder, the shoulder over the hip joint, and the hip joint over the lateral aspect of the ankle. This is a generalization, of course, but one that provides a baseline for discussion. When the upper body falls out of alignment with the hips and lower body, subtle accommodations are made by the body over time. An example would be an elderly person leaning forward resulting in shuffling of their feet rather than planting and pushing off with the ball of their foot. (Note: Certain medical conditions, such as Parkinson's disease or scoliosis, can cause complications with balance and posture).

## 10 TIPS FOR BETTER POSTURE

1. **Breathe deeply.** Proper technique is to breath into your belly five times, expanding your chest, ribs, belly and lower back. Stretch your arms and legs in all directions elongating all tissues at the neck, shoulders and hips. Squeeze your shoulder blades five times for 3 seconds.

2. **Use lumbar support for short periods of time when sitting.** A rolled-up towel can suffice, positioned at the lower back curvature. Reinforcing the natural lower back curve allows ease of function above and below the lower back.

3. **Adjust the height of your desk chair.** Ideally, your hips should be positioned above your knees. Assure your elbows are at or above the height of your wrists. Shoulder discomfort, neck pain, and even chronic conditions such as carpel tunnel syndrome can occur if left uncorrected.

4. **Use quick, easy-to-implement exercises.** Facing a wall, extend both arms above your head, positioning both hands flat on the wall. Descend into a squat as far as possible, sliding your hands down the wall. Try to feel this in your middle back and shoulders.

5. **Maintain good neck range of movement.** While sitting down, stretch your neck around to alleviate discomfort. Do this while tilting your chin down, ear to each side, and extending your head back, pushing your chin to the ceiling. Return to neutral between each position change, breathing out as you move into the stretch, and in as you return to neutral. Sit quietly before standing to prevent any dizziness.

6.  **Focus on doing more extensions.** These include planks (positional holds), lateral flexions and rotational exercises. Do fewer exercises that flex the spine (i.e. crunches).

7.  **Strengthen your core.** Exercises that involve lifting, weight shifting, directional changes, and slow, downward movements (like descending stairs) strengthen important core muscles used in daily activities. For example, when picking up anything from below your knees, drop your hips back while keeping your chest up. Keep whatever you're picking up close to the body as you stand up.

8.  **Strengthen areas important to good posture.** Building good posture starts from the ground up. Strengthening, stretching and massaging the tissues around the feet and ankles can ease standing and walking strain, particularly after a long day. Strengthen your arches by pulling a towel with your toes or slow controlled Calf/Shin Raise (Double Leg or Single Leg) on a step. Lengthen and soften the arch by rubbing a tennis ball or frozen tennis ball container from the big toe to heel.

9.  **Practice good hand flexibility.** Your hands are in a "curled position" most of the day. Stretch these muscles by pulling your hand into flexed and extended positions at least once an hour throughout the day.

10. **Keep a full range of motion in your hips.** This is an important factor to decreasing discomfort in the lower back. Try crossing your ankle over your opposite knee to stretch your hip, doing so for 1 minute per side.

---

**PARKINSON'S FIT TIP: EXTENSION VS. FLEXION EXERCISES**

Parkinson's disease may result in a forward postural lean. During walking, this position may lead to gait compensations such as shuffling. One approach to counter this forward position is by using extension exercises for the upper and lower body. Upper body exercises include back extensions and rows; lower body exercises include hip bridges and stationary lunges.

# CHAPTER 5

## Rules of the Road: Exercise Precautions

In the next chapter, you will find a series of exercises carefully selected to help people with Parkinson's retain as much normal function as possible. These exercises target improved mobility, increased flexibility, and strength training. The exercises and accompanying programs are designed to be safe and effective for people in varying stages of Parkinson's.

The programs outlined in Chapter 7 can be adapted to suit your unique needs and abilities. The best exercises are the ones that can be performed consistently over a number of years. In performing these exercises, you will be participating in a process called **motor learning**. In order to experience the benefits of physical activity, you must commit to regular exercise over an extended period of time.

It is important to remember that whenever you try something new, frustration is a natural part of the process. However, stress and frustration exacerbate the motor symptoms of Parkinson's disease, so you must be patient as you learn new physical and mental exercises.

The first few weeks of the program are called the **cognitive (or verbal) stage**, during which you will be developing a general understanding of what to do and how to do it. This stage generally lasts 3–4 weeks.

During the second stage, the **associative stage**, you will be able to perform the movements, but there may be some errors or flaws in your form. This stage usually lasts anywhere from 2–3 weeks.

The final stage, the **autonomous stage**, is when you are able to perform the exercises with proper technique and can repeat sets and reps week after week.

## EXERCISE ESSENTIALS CHECKLIST

### Exercise Preparation
- **Exercise location**: Is your environment safe, clean, and free from debris?
- **Proper footwear**: Are you wearing proper athletic footwear?
- **Comfortable athletic wear**: Do you have clothes that allow freedom of movement?
- **Hydration**: Be sure to drink 6–8 glasses of water during the course of your day.

### Exercise Equipment
- **Rolled-up towel**: Can be used for resistance training, balancing on the floor, etc.
- **Mirror**: Provides visual feedback on cueing and technique.
- **Dumbbells**: 5–10 pound range is generally appropriate.
- **TheraBand**: Light-colored bands offer less resistance and dark-colored bands offer more resistance.
- **Physioball**: Inflate the ball to the point where you can press your thumb on the surface without it sinking in.
- **Tennis ball or racquet ball**: For hand and foot therapy.

## IMPORTANT SAFETY PRECAUTIONS

In this section, you will find practical safety precautions to observe when exercising. Take the time to read them carefully and incorporate them into your routine. Please be advised that it is essential you see your healthcare provider regularly for check-ups, especially before beginning any new kind of fitness regimen.

**Body positioning**: Brace your core, achieve proper alignment, feel the placement of your feet, and always move from your core first before moving your limbs.

**Keep a health journal**: Record how you are feeling on any given day, along with the activities you did during that time. You should also record what kinds of exercises you did on each day, and how you felt both during and after your exercise session. Keeping track of this information will help you better understand your own health and track your progress.

**Rate of Perceived Exertion (RPE)**: You can use the chart below to gauge how hard you are working during your session. The corresponding numerical values may also be helpful for you to record in your health journal, should you choose to keep one. These values are included in the workout programs as an indicator of how much effort you should be expending in each routine.

| | |
|---|---|
| 1 | No Exertion at All |
| 2 | Extremely Light |
| 3 | Very Light |
| 4 | Moderate Light |
| 5 | Light |
| 6 | Moderate Hard |
| 7 | Hard (Heavy) |
| 8 | Very Hard |
| 9 | Extremely Hard |
| 10 | Full Exertion |

**Talk Test**: This is another useful way to determine how hard you are working. As you exercise, gauge how easily you are able to converse. If you can carry a conversation with ease while exercising, you are likely working aerobically, which means your body is using oxygen as its primary energy source. If you can work aerobically for 30–45 minutes, your body will begin using fat as an energy source, which is an excellent foundation for building your exercise program.

**Anaerobic Work**: Anaerobic work, characterized as medium intensity, should be introduced 8 weeks into your exercise program. Examples include hill walking, bike sprints, etc. When performing anaerobic exercise, you may notice your leg muscles starting to feel a bit tight; your chest will expand, you will begin to sweat, and your heart rate will reach about 40–50 beats above your resting heart rate.

### Adapting Your Home for Parkinson's Disease

**Daily Safety**: Wearing a fanny pack around your waist is always a good safety precaution when it includes a charged cell phone in addition to a printed list of important emergency contact phone numbers such as police, fire, family, and neighbors. Also put a copy on the fridge or in another easy to access place in the house.

**Bathroom**: Install grab bars and a sitting bench in the shower to keep steady while bathing. Add a rubber mat in the tub or shower to avoid slipping. Use non-skid bath mats on the floor.

**Kitchen**: Use plastic containers as opposed to glass to avoid breakage. Add non-skid rubber mats by the sink, dishwasher, and stove.

**Living areas**: Declutter your space for ease of movement, removing all accent and throw rugs that are easy to trip over. Wall to wall carpeting is best. Tie up any loose wires and electrical cords.

**Hallways and stairways**: Make sure halls, stairways, and entrances are well lit with overhead lights with light switches at the top and the bottom of the areas. Install railings on both sides of any stairs and near all doorknobs.

**Lighting**: Add nightlights in bathrooms, bedrooms and hallways or leave the overhead lights on at night. Make sure lamps and light switches are easy to reach from your bed as well.

## DETERMINING YOUR HEART RATE

To determine your heart rate, place the tips of your index, second and third fingers on your wrist, below the base of your thumb. You can also place the tips of your index and second fingers on your neck, along either side of your windpipe. During exercise, it is recommended that you find your pulse on your wrist, rather than on your neck.

When pressing lightly with your fingers, you should be able to feel your pulse. If you don't feel your pulse, move your fingers around slightly until you find it. Count the number of beats you feel in 10 seconds. Using that number, calculate your heart rate with the formula below:

**(Beats in 10 seconds) x 6 = (Heart rate)**

Adults over 18 years of age typically have a resting heart rate of 60–100 beats per minute. To better understand your own heart rate, you should check your pulse both before and immediately after exercising. This will give you a better idea of what your body normally does at rest, and what level your heart should be working at during an exercise session.

### Calculating Your Target Heart Rate

Your target heart rate is the level of exertion you should aim for when exercising in order to gain the most benefits from your workout. Your target heart rate is also a useful range for how your body is responding to exercise. Your target heart rate is 60–80 percent of your maximum heart rate, depending on what level of exertion you wish to work at.

## DIFFERENT TRAINING ZONES

Below is a list of the different levels of exertion and the corresponding percentage you would reference to determine your target heart rate. Please note, heart rate can be influenced by many different factors including sleep, stimulants, and stress. Keeping a record of your heart every few weeks combined with your RPE is a more well-rounded benchmark.

**Recovery Zone (60–70 percent).** Recovery training should fall into this zone (ideally at the lower end). It is also useful for very early pre-season and closed season cross-training when the body needs to recover and replenish.

**Aerobic Zone (70–80 percent).** Exercising in this zone will help develop your aerobic system and, in particular, your ability to transport and utilize oxygen. Continuous or rhythmic endurance training, like running and hiking, should fall in this heart rate zone.

**Anaerobic Zone (80–90 percent).** Training in this zone will help to improve your body's ability to deal with lactic acid. It may also help to increase your lactate threshold.

You can use the formulas below to calculate your maximum heart rate and then to find your target heart rate.

**220 – age = Maximum heart rate**

**(Maximum heart rate) x (training percentage) = Target heart rate**

For example, if a 50-year-old woman wishes to train at 70 percent of her maximum heart rate, she would use the below calculations:

**220 – 50 = 170**

**170 x 70% = 119**

She would thus aim to reach a heart rate of 119 during her exercise in order to work at her target heart rate.

## ASSESSMENT AND SCREENING

Before beginning any exercise program, it's important to establish a baseline. This baseline provides you with a foundation to interpret on-going feedback on your progress. Thankfully, the world of human movement science includes a seemingly endless variety of screenings, tests and evaluations that can provide useful data, tailored to a specific audience.

In the case of Parkinson's, the patient using this program is understood to have gone through an extensive medical exam with their primary care provider and neurologist, including recent blood lab results and a physical work up (including a sub max or maximal stress test). The results of these exams are what determine whether a patient is cleared for physical activity.

### Activities of Daily Living

We recognize our readers may have some limitations related to Parkinson's that make activities of daily living more challenging, while understanding there will be many readers exploring this resource for different roles—be it caregiver, loved one, or even a health professional. With that said, for those of our readers who may have physical limitations, it is important to establish benchmarks to measure improvement. Improvement is relative so don't get discouraged everyone can make strides by establishing a daily regimen.

Perform these movements as a baseline comparison for activities performed throughout your daily routine.

**Basic Activities of Daily Living (ADLs).** Basic ADLs are those tasks we perform on a daily basis. These tasks are generally self-care in nature. How many of the following can you complete without difficulty?

- Bathing
- Dressing
- Self-feeding
- Personal hygiene and grooming
- Toilet hygiene

**Instrumental Activities of Daily Living (IADLs).** Instrumental ADLs are slightly more complex uses of the body's functional mobility, and typically involve multiple basic ADLs being performed simultaneously. IADLs are relevant to Parkinson's treatment because of the way the disease affects muscle control, rigidity, and ultimately compensatory posture (i.e. forward lean) as a result of an altered gait pattern (think shuffling as compared to normal strides).

Postural conditions can impact one's ability to perform these activities. For example, the inability to raise one's arm above their head due to rounded shoulders or kyphosis prohibits one from being able to place dishes in a cabinet. Or, a limited ability to bend over (using proper squat mechanics) without low back pain makes it much more difficult to pick something up off of the floor.

> **PARKINSON'S FIT TIP:**
> **UPPER BODY AND MOVEMENT QUALITY**
> Movement quality is the degree to which someone can execute basic human movements with precision and repetition. For example, take walking: walking requires a certain level of coordination between the upper and lower body. Those afflicted with Parkinson's experience rigidity and contractures in the muscles around the shoulder girdle, the result of which can be a shortened arm swing and gait to better increase their stability during walking. This results in the common Parkinson's trait known as shuffling. To improve this, flexibility exercises focusing on the neck, shoulders and chest should be performed regularly.

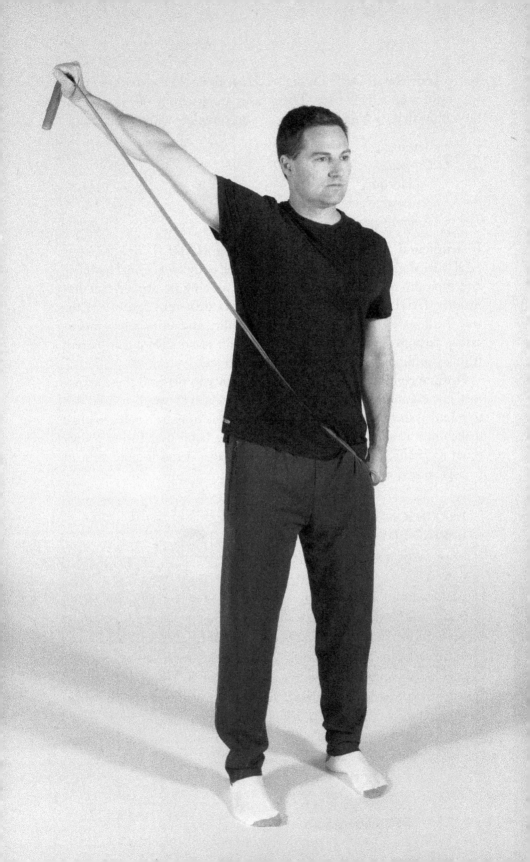

# CHAPTER 6

# The Exercises

I n selecting the perfect exercises to aid in both general and targeted Parkinson's improvement, adopting a comprehensive movement approach is paramount. The exercises featured in this book take into account the fact that Parkinson's disease is a condition where movement quality deteriorates over time.

These exercises were purposely selected with an eye towards balancing all three planes of movement: frontal (side to side), sagittal (front to back), and transverse (rotational). By working these planes individually or in combination, we allow for a never-ending selection of program possibilities, as well as countless exercises to choose from.

The concept of exercise relies on structure, and for good reason: there are specific techniques and forms necessary to perform each movement correctly. That being said, there is also a fun, unstructured aspect to daily movement that allows us to express ourselves in ways a machine, dumbbell, or TheraBand could never accomplish.

**A list of healthy activities that can improve movement, balance and mobility includes:**

- Walking outside or in a mall (navigating obstacles, people and stairs)
- Dancing
- Yoga classes
- Tai chi classes
- Stepping over obstacles
- Marching to music with big arm swings
- Sports (ping pong, golf, tennis, volleyball)
- Aerobic/Jazzercise classes

## HOW DID WE CHOOSE OUR EXERCISES?

**We selected exercises based on three straightforward principles:**

1. **Keep it simple.** We selected movements that require a minimal amount of fitness experience, with an easy learning curve.
2. **Address disease concerns.** We selected movements that address the physical aspect of Parkinson's, first and foremost.
3. **Minimal equipment.** This book assumes readers have limited access to equipment and facilities.

**In terms of specifically addressing Parkinson's-specific fitness concerns, we focus on:**

- Improving upper body range of motion during stride
- Improving lower body range of motion during stride
- Enhancing overall control, including change of direction, stopping, starting
- Strengthening postural muscles
- Addressing contractures using hold and relax stretching
- Progressing from static to dynamic exercises when tolerated

## BENCHMARKS

Our benchmarks are practical. We establish three categories of assessment that cast a wide net, related to Parkinson's.

**Our assessment categories are as follows:**

**Mobility**. Mobility is a general term covering flexibility, balance, and general body control. As we age, it's generally thought that our movement quality decreases due to loss of muscle strength, toning and slowing of reflexive response. Fortunately, through healthy living movement quality can be relatively maintained. In respect to Parkinson's, a degenerative condition that affects the mind and body, independent activities will still become increasingly difficult as a person's quality of movement degrades. This is why it's important to do what you can, while you can, to ensure any decline remains gradual.

**Physical**. Physical benchmarking means establishing clear markers for strength and endurance. Improvements in this category trickle over into the mobility and activities of daily living assessments. Building strength tends to produce positives changes in body composition, toning, and reflexes.

**Activities of Daily Living (ADLs)**. ADLs are activities we perform every day, regardless of age, gender, physical status, or occupation. Your Parkinson's program is only as effective as the degree to which it supports positive lifestyle changes related to your condition.

---

**PARKINSON'S FIT TIP: POSTURE SELF-ASSESSMENT SCREEN**

A simple assessment, called 3 Points of Contact, can be used to establish a personalized spinal baseline, utilizing three distinct points of contact: the head, the middle back and the pelvis.

To perform this screen, align a broomstick along your spine. Your three points should be in contact with the broomstick, going from head to middle spine to sacrum.

---

## STABILITY VS. MOBILITY

A few things to bear in mind, given the importance we'll be placing on mobility and range of movement in this program. The body's movements consist of alternating patterns of "stability and mobility." By design, joints have primary actions such as hinging, rotation, and flexion. Corresponding to the action is their innate action for stability or mobility.

**Below are some examples, as well as the category they traditionally fall under:**

- **Feet**: Stability. Feet support the load of the body.
- **Ankles**: Mobile. Ankles move forward and backward to propel the body.
- **Knees**: Stability. Knees act as a stable connector to the major bones above and below. They assist in supporting the load of the body by their location in the lower extremity.
- **Hips**: Mobility.
- **Lower Spine**: Stability.

## THE EXERCISES

The following section presents each exercise featured in this book's program. The description for each exercise looks to provide a detailed understanding of how to perform the given exercise. Each exercise also includes a "Feel It Here" note, indicating where in your body you should most feel the effects of the movement.

# Overhead Squat
## FEEL IT HERE: Legs, Hips, Middle Spine, Shoulders

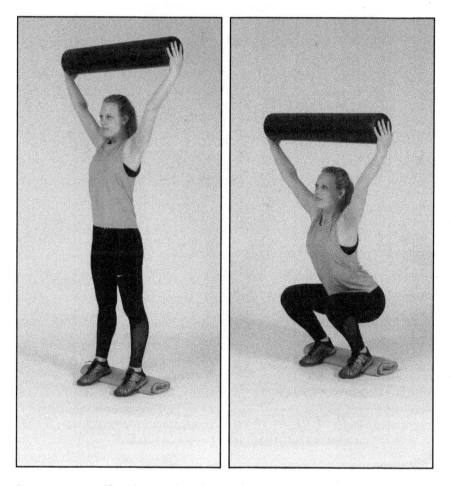

Position yourself with your feet hip-width apart. Point your toes at the 11 and 1 o'clock positions respectively, as this will allow your hips, knees, and ankles to move together properly during the squatting movement. Place a dowel (or broomstick) on the crown of your head so your elbows are at a 90-degree angle, then press the stick above your head. Place a half roller under your heels if you feel your body pitching forward. Drop your hips as low as possible.

# Standing with Eyes Closed
## FEEL IT HERE: General Body Awareness

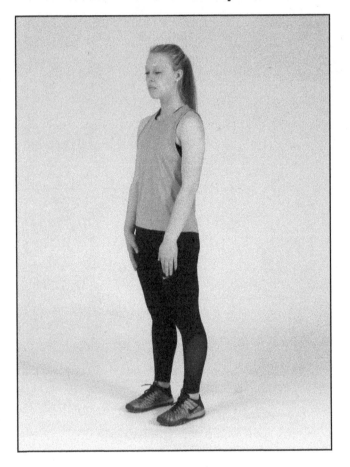

Stand with your feet hip-width apart. You should stand near a wall or partner for safety. For the two-legged test, rest your hands at your side and close your eyes. With both feet on the ground, feel a natural sway similar to a tree in the wind. For the one-legged test, close your eyes once your foot is off the ground. With one foot on the ground the sway will increase dramatically with your body wanting to make very quick readjustments to stabilize.

# Push-ups

## FEEL IT HERE: **Chest, Shoulders, Mid-section**

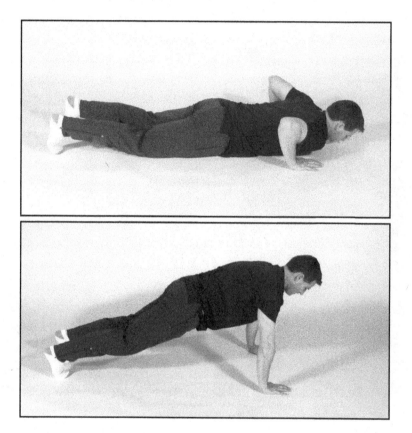

Position yourself on your stomach. Your hands should be parallel to your shoulders. Place a dowel stick along the spine so contact is made with your head and sacrum. Begin the movement by bracing your stomach. Push your toes and hands into the floor, then attempt to press your body away from the floor until your elbows are straight. You should feel your shoulder blades come together as you return to your starting position.

# Wall Sit with Foam Roller
## FEEL IT HERE: Legs, Hips

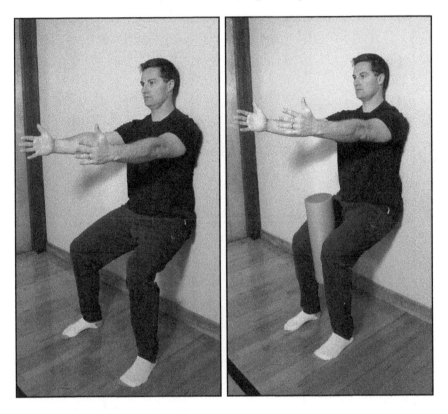

With your feet and knees hip-width apart, squeeze the foam roller between the knees. Keep your hips and shoulders against a wall. Hold the position.

# Dumbbell Row (Double Arm)
## FEEL IT HERE: Arm, Shoulder, Back

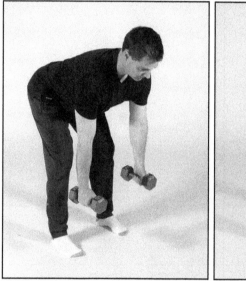 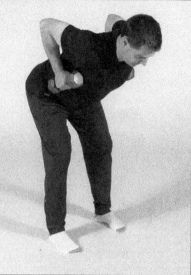

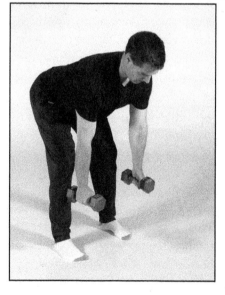

Either kneel (and use one arm) or stand and use both arms, shown above. Perform a row, pulling your elbows behind your back and then extend your arm fully in back of you to work the triceps.

# Deadlift (Double Leg or Single Leg)
## FEEL IT HERE: Legs, Hips, Mid-section

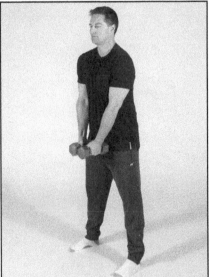

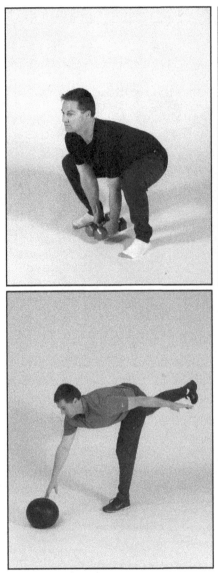

With your feet hip to shoulder-width apart and arms extended downward grabbing the barbell or dumbbell, press your feet into the floor, brace your stomach, and begin the upward ascent. Breathe out on the exertion or upward movement, pausing at the top. Begin the downward movement with the hips first, showing the chest forward.

Modifications for this exercise can be done by starting the bar from a higher position on boxes or benches. The single leg version involves one foot staying on the ground, with the opposite foot raising up behind the body until it is parallel with the floor.

# Lateral Plank

**FEEL IT HERE: Shoulder, Mid-section, Hip**

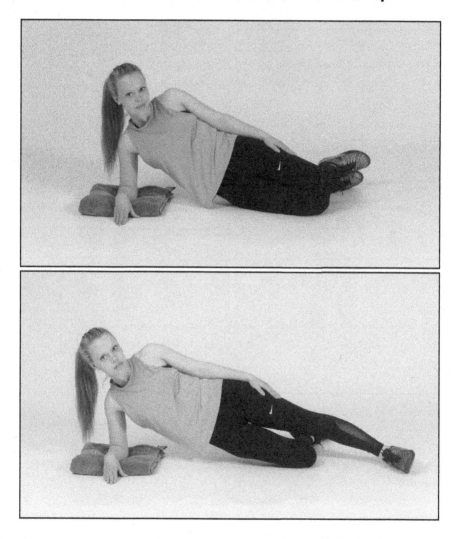

Position your body on one side, on your elbow and hip. Contract the side of your stomach and elevate your hip into alignment with the shoulders and knees.

# Hip Hinging
### FEEL IT HERE: Hip, Back

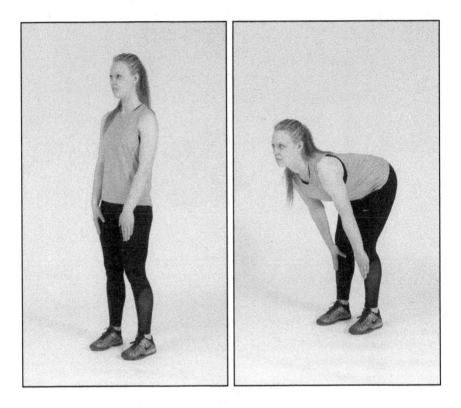

Start the squatting movement from your hips, letting the other parts follow. Feel your upper body positioned over the upper thighs as you bend during the downward motion. Brace your stomach, then begin the upward movement by pressing your feet into the floor, followed by pushing your hips through. For added help with stability, place a broomstick along your spine. Contact should be felt on the back of your head, middle back and tailbone.

# Spinal Whip

## FEEL IT HERE: Back, Mid-section

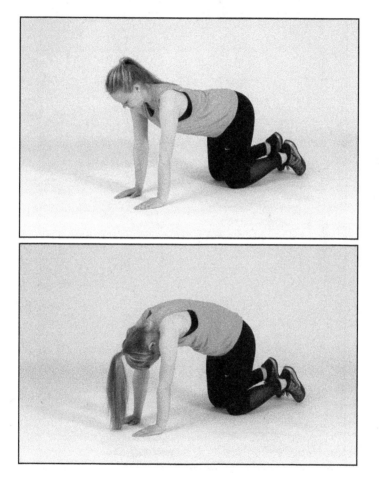

Begin on all fours or standing with your hands on your knees. Rotate from the shoulder blades as they move to the outside of the upper body. Emphasize moving from the middle back through the sternum.

# Shoulder Circles

## FEEL IT HERE: Shoulders, Arms

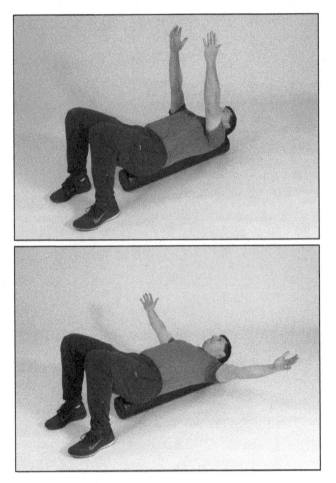

Lay down on the roller with your spine resting in the long position. If you need increased balance during the movement use a half roller or rolled up towel. Feel pressure on your spine. Only your head, middle back, and pelvis should be resting in contact with the roller. Initiate smooth circles with your arms as if you have a dinner tray in each hand.

# Thoracic Flex

## FEEL IT HERE: Mid-section

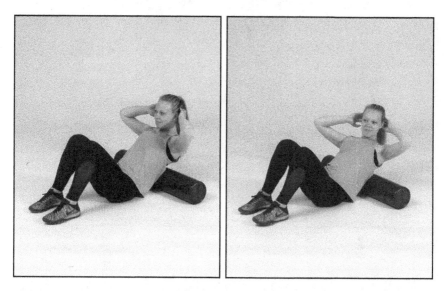

You can use a full roller, half roller, or thick, rolled up towel. Position the roller immediately below your shoulder blades. Your elbows should be pointed to the sides. Feel the foam roller pressing against your middle spine. Keep your ribs heavy into the ground so the core muscles are active and working through the entire motion. Your front abs will be working the entire time but the latter muscles, namely the obliques, are the actual movers.

# Cranial Release
## FEEL IT HERE: Neck, Head

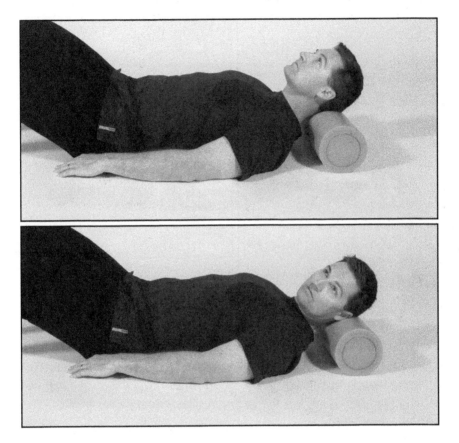

Lay on your back. Position the back of your head, right where it meets the base of your neck, on the roller. You should be in a comfortable position; draw your feet into your hips if needed. Your hands should be relaxed near the sides of your hips. If you need to stabilize the roller, place your hands on the sides of the roller. Rotate your head to the right and left. When rotating your head to the right and left, feel the small space that sits on either side of your head. Keep pressure in the roller by slightly extending your neck, emphasizing proper alignment.

# Scissor Stretch
## FEEL IT HERE: Legs, Hips

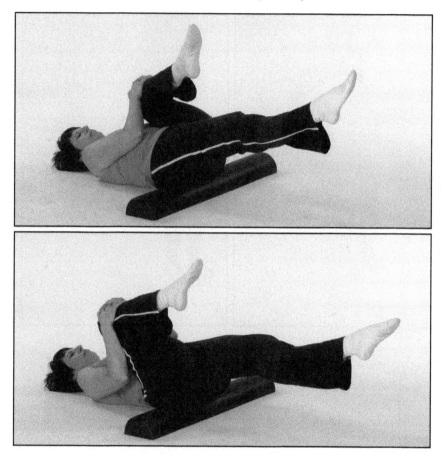

Lay on your back with your knees bent and feet close to your hips. Press your feet into the floor, then elevate your hips. Slide a foam roller (or very thick towel) beneath your tailbone/sacrum. Keeping your ribs heavy, pull one knee to your chest and hold. Extend the leg next, keeping ribs heavy, engaging the core. The sacrum is the flattish bone that positions itself directly below the lower back. Place the palm of your hand on the sacrum; it should fit nicely. The roller sits between the lower back and sacrum.

# Alphabet Series: T
### FEEL IT HERE: Chest, Back

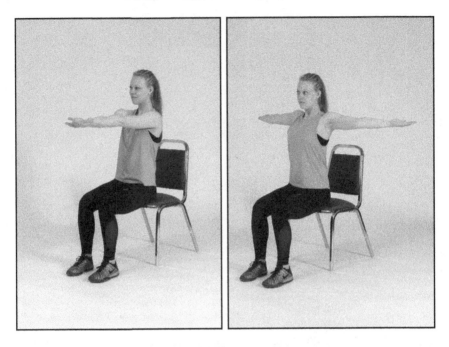

Sit upright on a sturdy surface. Squeeze your shoulder blades back and down. Draw both arms out from the mid-line of the body with palms up.

# Alphabet Series: Y

**FEEL IT HERE: Arms, Upper Back, Middle Back**

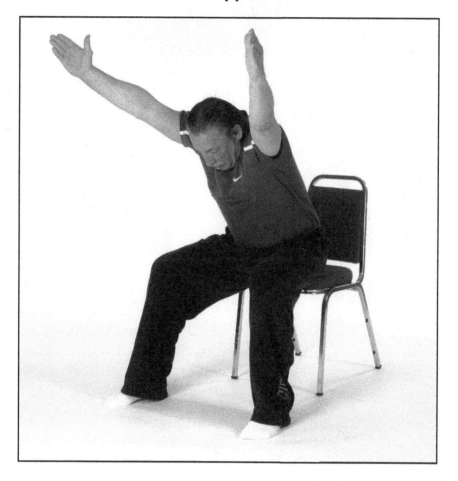

Sit upright on a sturdy surface. Squeeze your shoulder blades back and down. Draw both arms up, and straight out in front of your body at a 45-degree angle

# Alphabet Series: W

### FEEL IT HERE: Arms, Shoulders, Upper Back, Middle Back

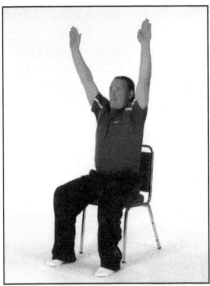

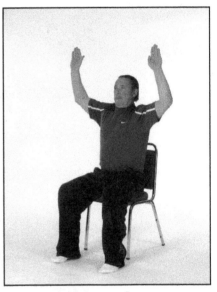

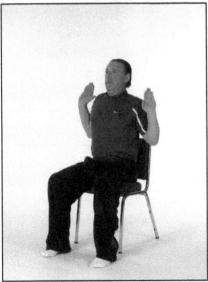

Sit upright on a sturdy surface. Squeeze your shoulder blades back and down. Draw both elbows down and back into the middle spine. Hold, then release.

# Ribcage Opener
## FEEL IT HERE: Shoulders, Mid-section

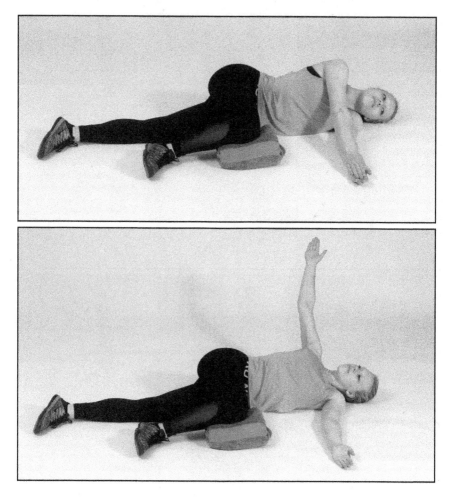

Lay on the ground and position a rolled-up towel or foam roller under your knee. Start with your hands together. Press your knees into the object then initiate rotation with your hand. Follow the rotation down the arm until you feel it through your ribcage.

# Ankle Pumps
## FEEL IT HERE: Ankles, Shin, Calf

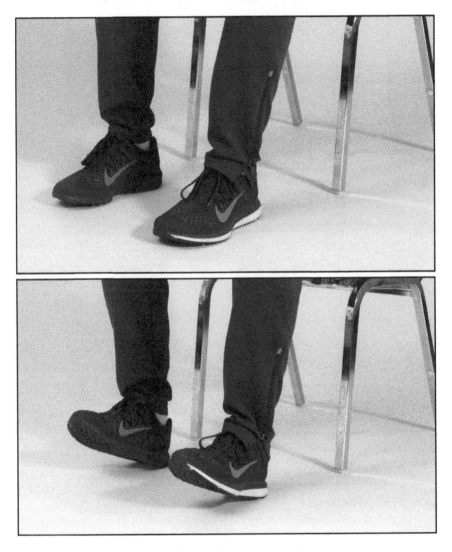

Gently point and flex the foot, reaching out through the front of the big toe. Pull the toes back by pushing through the heel.

# Rotational Chair Stretch
## FEEL IT HERE: Mid-section

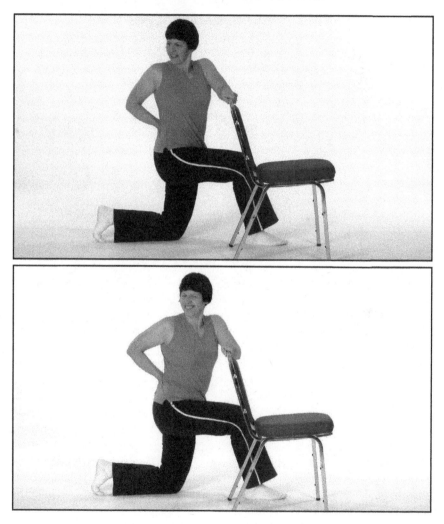

Begin on one knee, behind and to the side of a chair, with one hand on the back of the chair for support, as show above. Place your other hand on your back to use as leverage in order to achieve greater rotation. Take a deep breath in, then rotate as shown above.

# Calf/Shin Raise
## (Double Leg or Single Leg)
### FEEL IT HERE: Calves, Legs

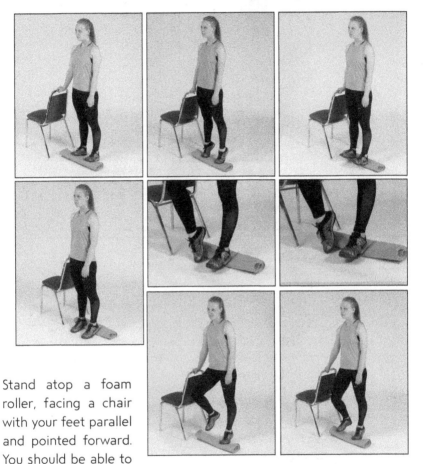

Stand atop a foam roller, facing a chair with your feet parallel and pointed forward. You should be able to see the front of your feet when looking down. Keep your hands light against the chair. Begin by pressing the balls of your feet into the ground, then pull your heels up towards the back of your hips. To increase the effort on the calves and feet, perform the movement higher off the ground and on a single leg.

# Heel to Toe Rocks

## FEEL IT HERE: Feet, Calves,

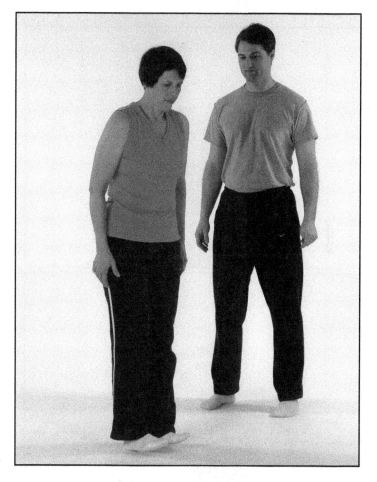

Partner rocks back and forth from the toes to heels as you provide support if needed.

# Band Pull-Aparts
### FEEL IT HERE: Arms, Upper Back

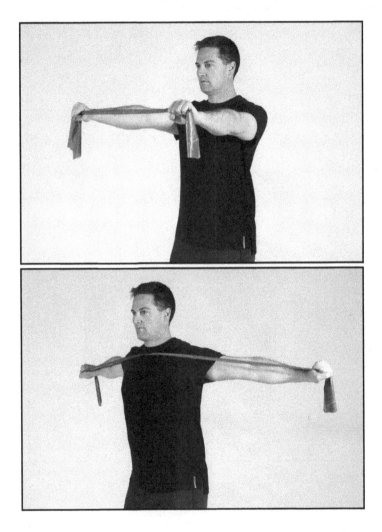

Keep the weight of your body in the feet and hips by slightly leaning forward. This allows the shoulders and arms to move naturally. Cue the shoulder blades to stay back and down thereby relaxing the upper neck muscles.

# Band Rows

## FEEL IT HERE: Arms, Shoulders

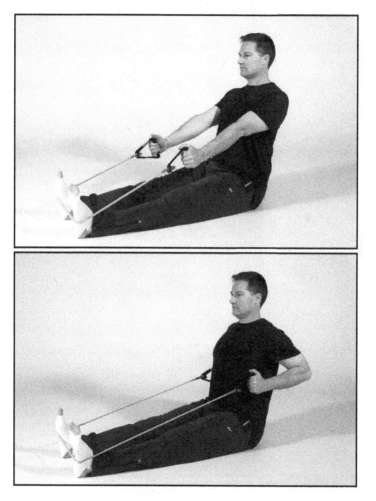

Position your body in an upright position on either a ball or bench. First, pull your shoulder blades back. Keeping them back, pull one elbow back at a time. Keep your ribs heavy and core contracted during each pressing repetition. Breathe out during each rep and breathe in upon return to the starting position. This exercise can also be done while standing.

# Band Presses (Alternating)

## FEEL IT HERE: Chest, Shoulders, Arms

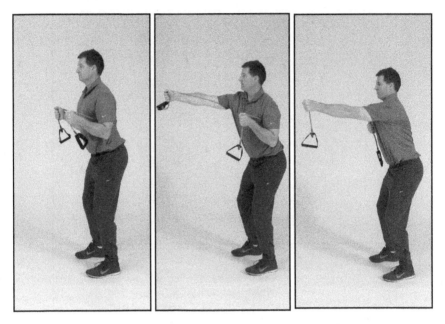

Position your body in a standing position in a normal stance or a split stance. Press your hands out in front until your elbows are fully extended. Keep the ribs heavy and core contracted during each pressing repetition. Breathe out during each extension and breathe in upon return to the starting position. This exercise can also be done while in an upright position (shown above) or while sitting on either a ball or bench on either a ball or a bench.

# Towel Pulls

### FEEL IT HERE: Feet

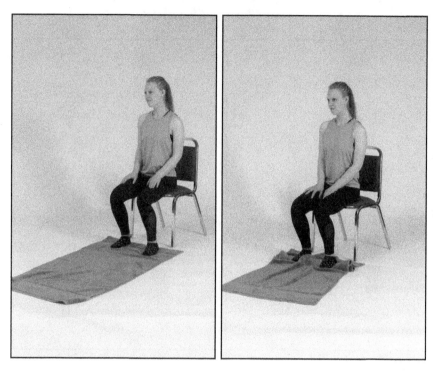

Take your shoes off. Lay a large towel flat on the floor. Pull the towel into the foot using the toes and arch, as shown. For added resistance, place a small weight on the towel.

# Chest Stretch
## (Open Arms) with Partner
### FEEL IT HERE: Chest, Shoulders, Arms

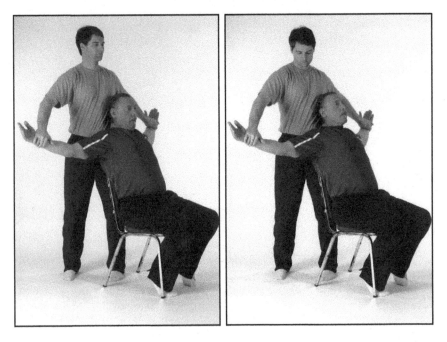

Stand behind your partner with your hands gently placed upon his or her upper arms. Keep your body positioned along your partner's spine to stabilize and assist in creating a greater stretch through the front of your partner's body.

# Partner Stability Pushes:
## Sitting and Standing
### FEEL IT HERE: Mid-section, Upper Body

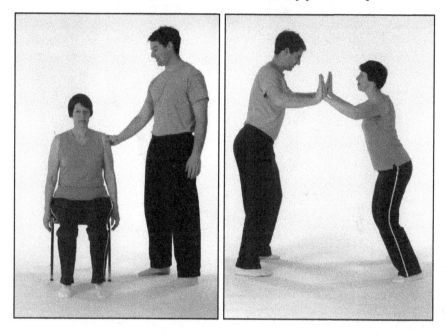

Your partner will start in a seated position. Instruct him or her to breathe during the entire exercise. Proceed to gently push at the shoulders, middle back, and front of the body. Once your partner feels comfortable with the seated position, try the standing position. Push your partner in the same spots.

# Weight Shifting
## FEEL IT HERE: Hips, Legs

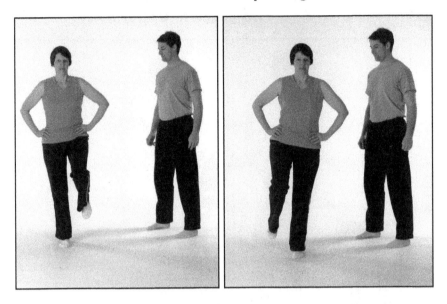

Your partner begins in normal walking position. As he or she walks forward, spot from the left to right leg, as your partner balances momentarily on each leg. Partner should feel the hips and legs working to stabilize the body during the momentary pause phase.

# Glute Bridge

## FEEL IT HERE: Legs, Hips, Back

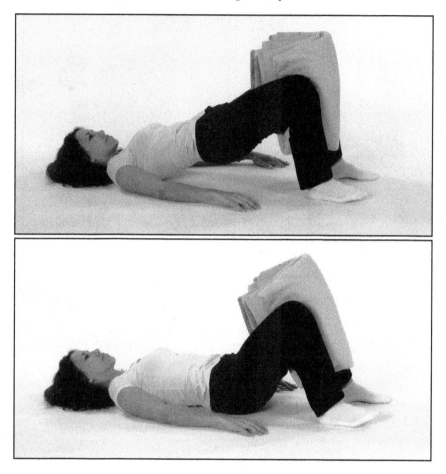

Lying supine with your knees bent and feet flat on the floor, contract your glutes and raise your hips off the floor until your body is in a straight line. Perform 1–3 sets of 10–15 repetitions.

Progress to a Single Leg Hip Bridge, then to performing the bridging action with feet on a physio/stability ball.

# Single Arm Dumbbell Row
## FEEL IT HERE: Shoulder, Arm

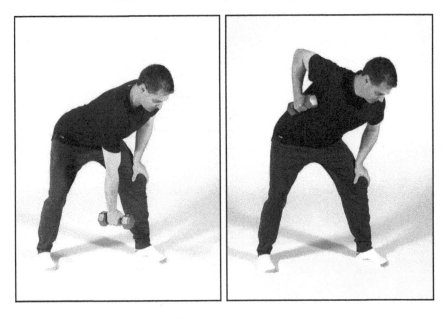

Grab a dumbbell and assume a deadlift position (lower back neutral, bent over at the waist, knees slightly bent). Place the hand without a dumbbell on your hip. Initiate the exercise by pulling your shoulder blades down and back while pulling the dumbbell up, keeping the elbow close to your body. Using only one dumbbell forces the body to use more core stability to maintain proper form.

# Stationary Lunge/Split Squat
## FEEL IT HERE: Legs, Hips

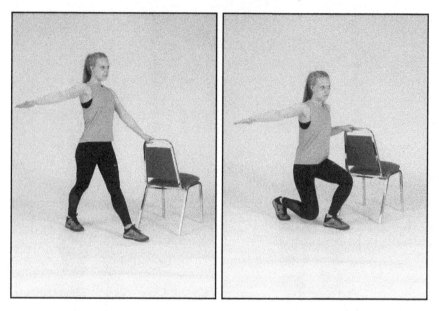

Assume a half-kneeling position with your right knee down and left knee up. Keeping your chest up and your shoulder blades pulled down and back (as though you were trying to put your shoulder blades into your back pocket), initiate the exercise by driving your left heel into the ground to push your hips up until your left leg is fully extended. Finish the movement by bending your left knee to lower yourself into a squatting position, until your right knee lightly taps the floor. You may hold onto an anchor point for balance, if needed.

# Draw the Sword

### FEEL IT HERE: Shoulder, Back

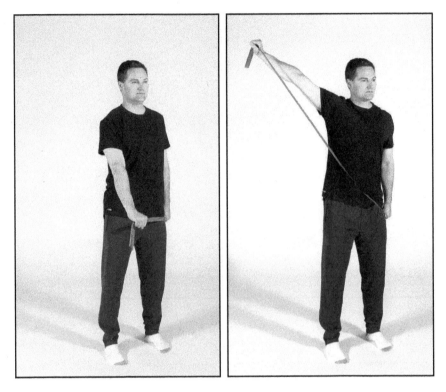

Perform this exercise sitting or standing. Reach across the body—palm down—to the opposite pocket. Imagine that you are pulling a sword and drawing it across your body. Rotate the hand and shoulder as your arm moves to the ending position, palm facing up.

# Back to Back Butterfly Stretch
## FEEL IT HERE: Hips, Groin

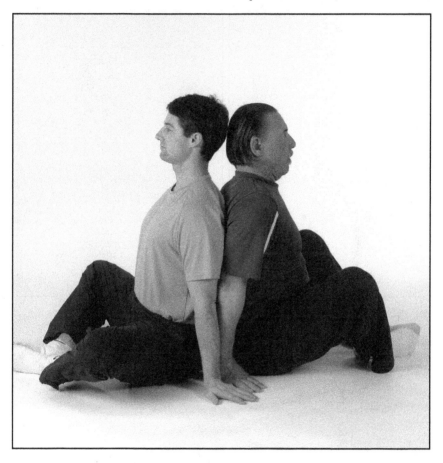

Sit back to back with your partner, and gently press your knees down.

# Chin Tuck

### FEEL IT HERE: Neck

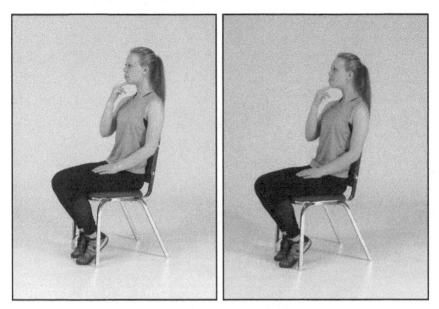

Sitting upright, gently press your chin backwards.

# Cobra

## FEEL IT HERE: Hips, Back

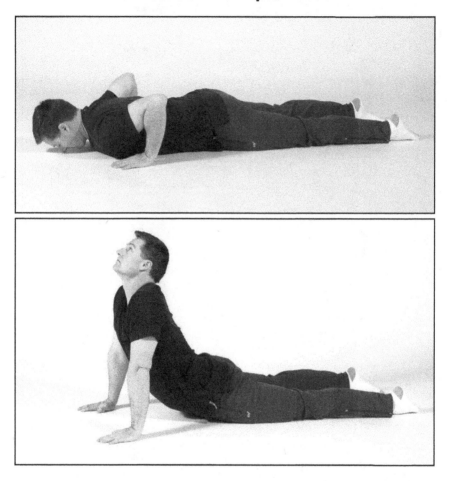

Starting on your stomach, breathe out and gently press upwards.

# Forward Plank

## FEEL IT HERE: Stomach, Hips

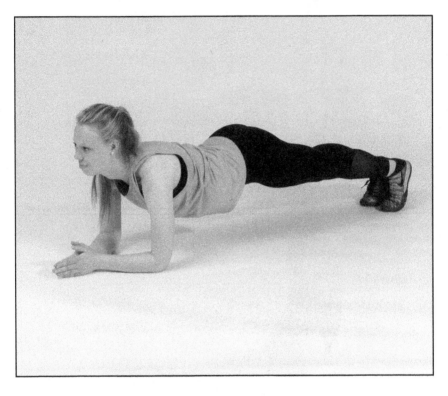

Begin on the floor, facing down. Press your palms together and your toes into the floor. Attempt to pull your upper back towards the ceiling, allowing the shoulder blades to move forward.

# Single Leg Hamstring Lifts

## FEEL IT HERE: Top of Foot, Back of Leg

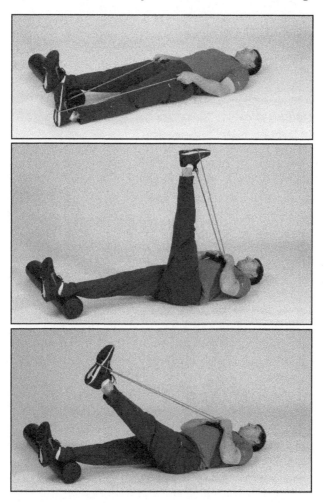

Lay on your back and wrap a stretch cord or fitness band around the arch of your foot. Pull your foot toward you, without letting your hip move. Hold the pressure for five seconds. Release and breathe out slowly. Repeat the movement in reverse from this position.

# Kegels

**FEEL IT HERE: Pelvis, Stomach, Hips**

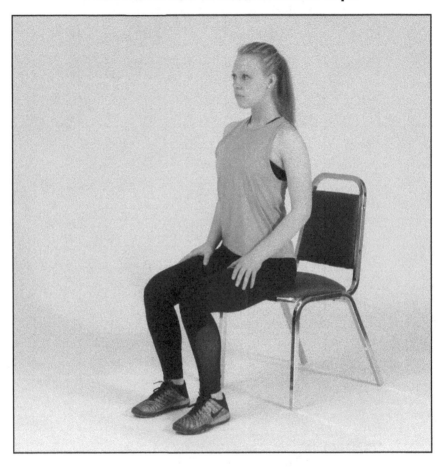

Begin by sitting on a physioball or chair. Pull your pelvic floor up and hold position.

# Hip Roller
## FEEL IT HERE: Hip

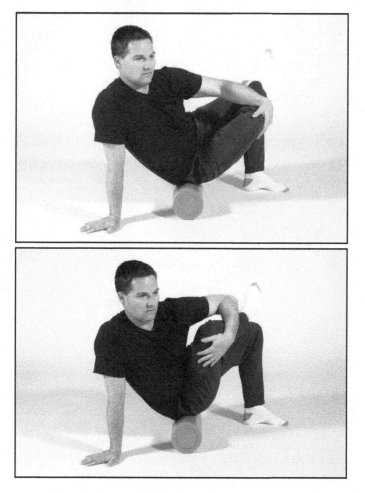

Start by sitting on the foam roller on the side of the hip you plan on rolling. Cross the same side's ankle over the opposite side's knee, until you feel the pressure in your hip.

# Quad Roller

### FEEL IT HERE: Upper Legs

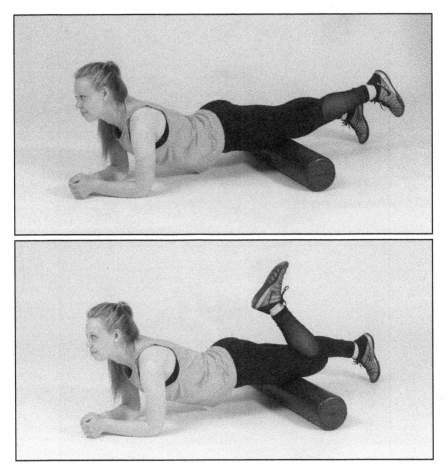

Start by positioning the foam roller on the front of the thighs. Keep your core braced. Flex and extend one knee at a time, moving to the next point on the thigh.

# Thoracic Spine Roller
## FEEL IT HERE: Middle Back, Upper Back

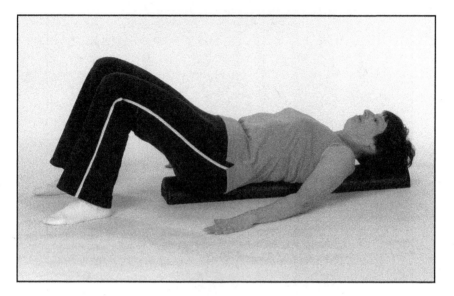

Start by positioning the foam roller on your back, just off center from the spine. Don't roll directly on the spine, but just off to the left or right. Don't roll the lower back near the lower ribs.

# Foot Taps

### FEEL IT HERE: Shins

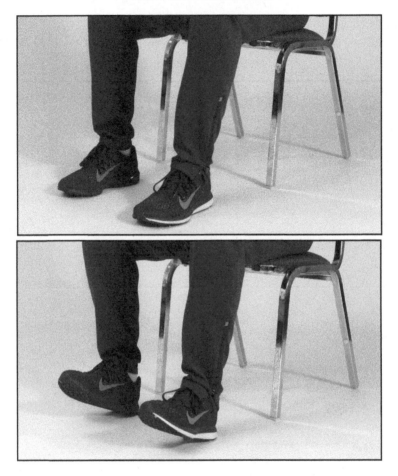

Begin in a sitting position towards the end of a chair. Tap your toes up and down together as quickly as possible, keeping your heels on the floor.

# Prayer Pose

### FEEL IT HERE: Back, Shoulder

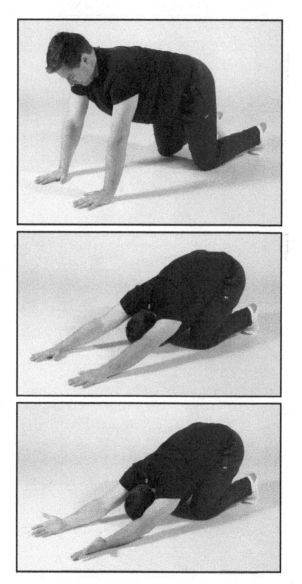

Begin in a kneeling position and reach through under the opposite side.

# All 4s

## FEEL IT HERE: Shoulders, Core, Legs

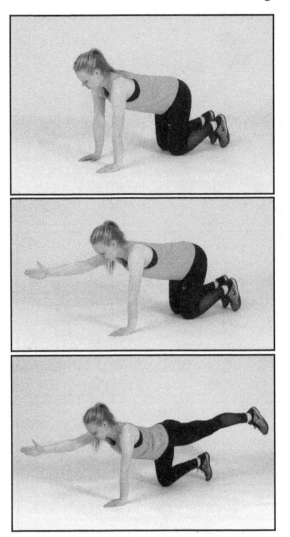

Starting on all fours, extend your opposite arm and leg, stabilizing with the hand and knee on the ground. Hold this extended position, then return to neutral.

# Deadbug

**FEEL IT HERE: Core**

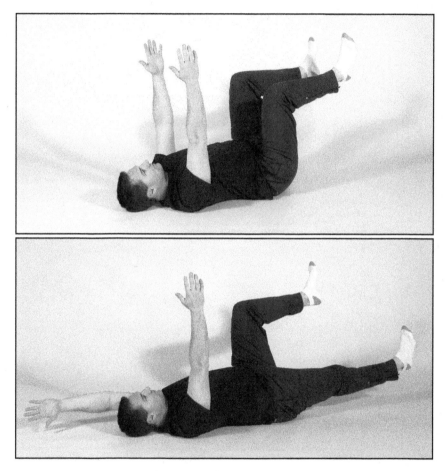

Starting on your back, begin with arms straight in front and knees bent over at the hips. Extend one arm, adding the opposite leg if you can keep your back from arching. Repeat sequence on other side.

# Supermans

### FEEL IT HERE: Back, Legs

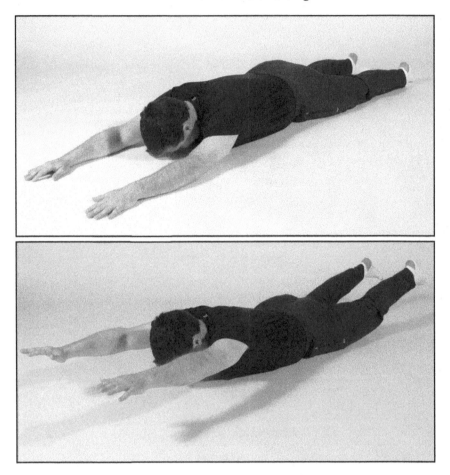

Starting on your stomach, extend your upper body off the ground. Hold this position, then return to the starting position. If you can complete this while maintaining control, repeat the sequence by lifting the upper body and legs off the ground.

# Ribs Heavy

## FEEL IT HERE: Lower Ribs, Abs

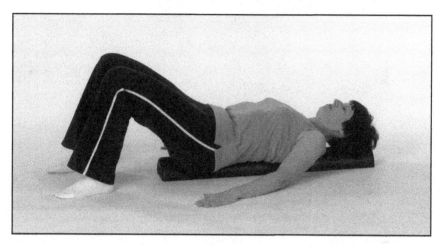

Use a foam roller or towel rolled up lengthwise. Make sure your head, middle back, and hips are in contact with the roller or towel. Feel your lower ribs make contact with the roller, yet make sure you have space in your lower back. This movement replaces pushing your lower back into the ground or flattening out your lower back during core movements, and will be applied to all exercises. When lying on your back, the body should contact the floor at your head, shoulders, hips, upper legs and calves. Your neck, lower back, and space behind your knees should be off the floor.

# Prone Extension

## FEEL IT HERE: Middle of Back, Lower Back, Hips

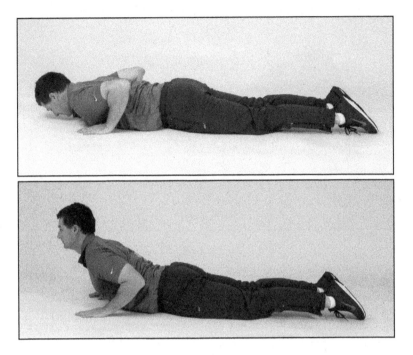

Lay face down, positioning your hands, palms down, against your forehead. Keep your head in light contact with your hands and lift from your middle back one vertebrae at a time.

# Sitting Hip Stretch
## FEEL IT HERE: Groin, Hips

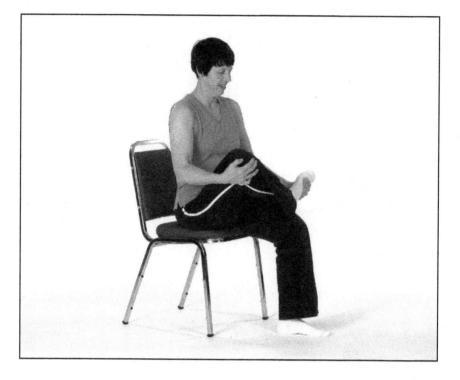

Sit upright with your hips at the same height as the knees. Breathe out and release the pressure. Pause, then assist the knees out farther. For additional support, sit against a chair back. Make sure the non-stretching hip stays firmly planted in the seat.

# Clock Lunge

### FEEL IT HERE: Hips, Legs

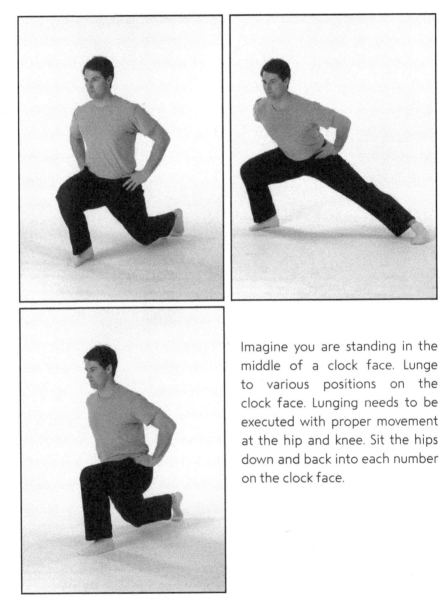

Imagine you are standing in the middle of a clock face. Lunge to various positions on the clock face. Lunging needs to be executed with proper movement at the hip and knee. Sit the hips down and back into each number on the clock face.

# Standing Single Arm Chest Press
## FEEL IT HERE: Chest, Shoulders, Arms

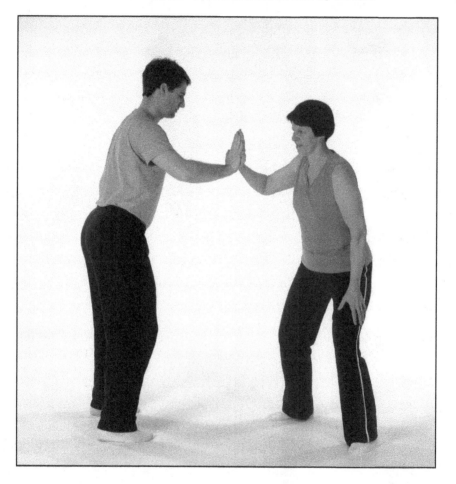

Using only one arm, press the palms of your hands against your partner's. Press the hands back and forth, resisting one another, but still allowing for range of motion similar to a dumbbell chest press. Be careful not to push your partner's arm too hard and be sure to stabilize forward and backward through your core.

# Standing Double Arm Chest Press

## FEEL IT HERE: Chest, Arms, Core

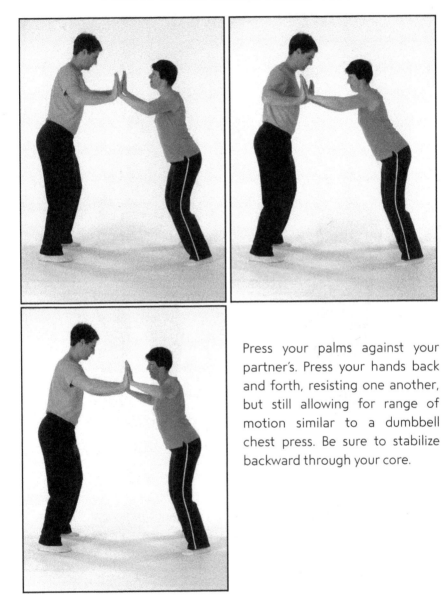

Press your palms against your partner's. Press your hands back and forth, resisting one another, but still allowing for range of motion similar to a dumbbell chest press. Be sure to stabilize backward through your core.

# Dumbbell Squat

## FEEL IT HERE: Core, Hips, Legs

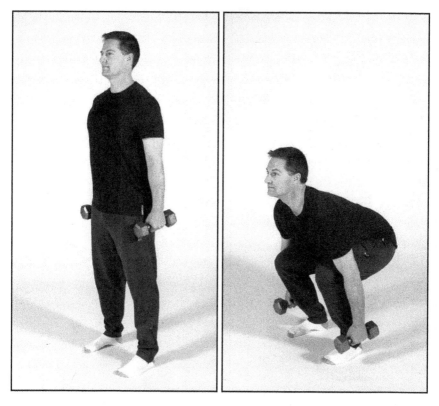

Extend two dumbbells above your head and stabilize. Squat to your lowest depth while maintaining a neutral spine, knees over the outside threes toes, and as a vertical shin as possible. Once you have reached a safe depth, drive your feet into the ground, keep your chest up and push your hips forward.

# Dumbbell Squat with Reach Across
## FEEL IT HERE: Core, Hips, Legs

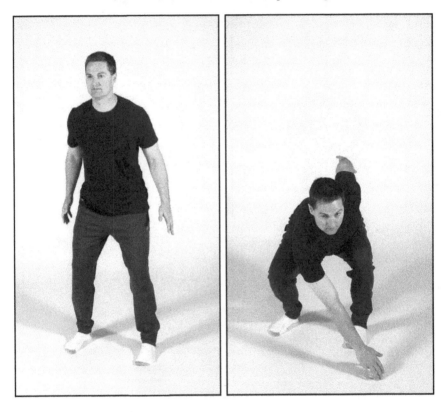

Keeping your arms raised and extended in front of your eyes, stand with your feet about shoulder width apart and toes straight ahead. Initiate the exercise by pushing your hips back with a neutral lower back, allowing your knees to bend naturally. Attempt to maintain a vertical shin as you squat down and pause for 2 seconds. Drive your heels into the ground to push yourself back up.

# Double Leg Deadlifts
## FEEL IT HERE: Legs, Hips, Core

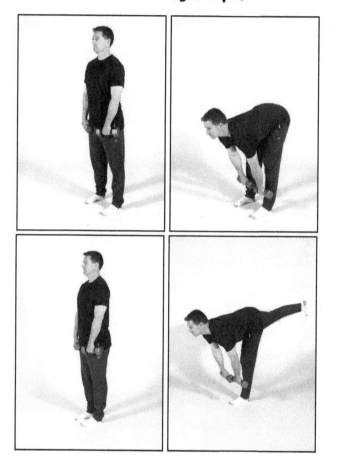

Standing up tall on one leg, place your hands on your hips and slightly bend your knees. Initiate the exercise by kicking your balance leg back until you feel a good stretch in the hamstring of the leg on the floor.

You may use an anchor point for your hands if you are having trouble balancing or if you want to emphasize stretching over balance. This variation of the movement places additional focus on the hamstrings.

# Abductor Stretch

## FEEL IT HERE: Outer Hip, Obliques, Lower Back

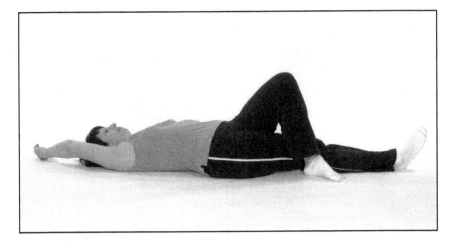

Keeping the non-stretching leg down on the floor, cross the opposite ankle over the leg, pressing against the knee. Hold the pressure for five seconds. Release and breathe out slowly. Repeat the movement from the newly obtained position.

# Band Pulls with One Knee Up
## FEEL IT HERE: Core, Arms, Chest, Legs

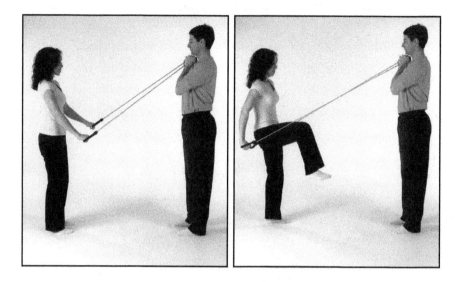

In a standing position, pull your knee upward towards your chest while pulling the arms to the sides of your body. Keep your ribs heavy and core contracted during each pressing repetition. Breathe out during each pressing rep and breathe in upon returning to the starting position.

# Windshield Washer
## FEEL IT HERE: Inner Hip Joints

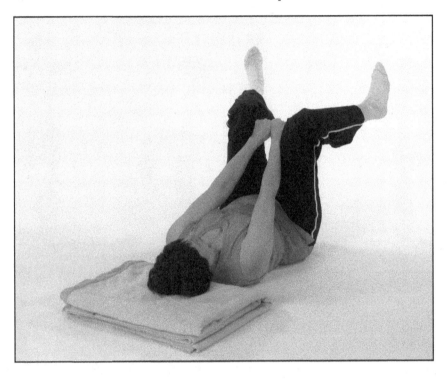

Lay on your back. Squeeze a ball or double fists between your knees. Position your head on a towel to take stress off your neck and arms. Maintain pressure on the object while rotating your hips inward.

# Band Pulls

## FEEL IT HERE: Arms, Back, Core

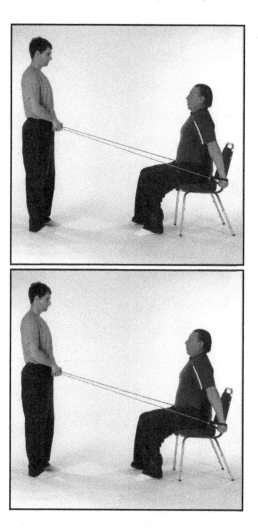

Keep the weight of your body in the feet and hips by slightly leaning forward. This allows the shoulders and arms to move naturally. Cue the shoulder blades to stay back and down thereby relaxing the upper neck muscles.

# Curling and Pressing Combo
## FEEL IT HERE: Arms, Shoulders

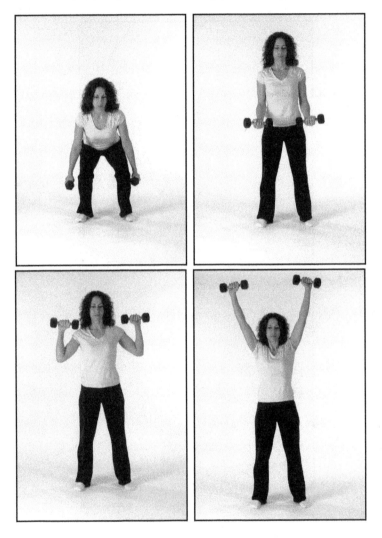

Position yourself in a half-squat position. Dumbbells should be by the sides of your body. Brace your core. Curl the dumbbells up first and then, press them above your head, keeping your shoulders in a neutral position.

# Hip Lifters
## FEEL IT HERE: Hips, Back

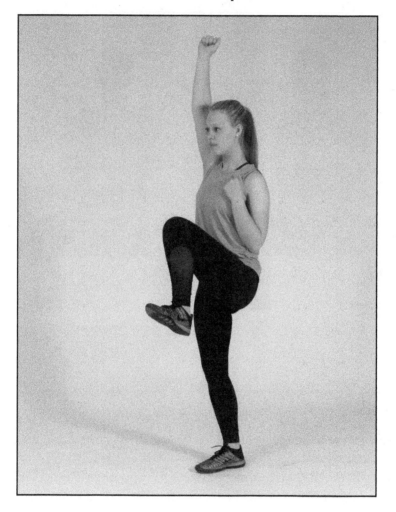

With elbows at your sides, draw the knee up and straighten arm to enhance balance. Pause in a single leg stance and return to starting stance. Feel the hips and back working throughout this exercise.

# Lateral Neck Stretch

### FEEL IT HERE: Neck, Shoulder

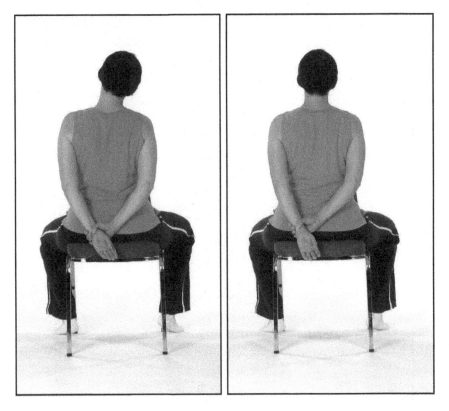

Sit with the arm of the shoulder to be stretched placed behind you. Gently drop your ear to your other shoulder. Then, grab the wrist of the shoulder/neck area being stretched. Relax the opposite side shoulder by breathing deeply into the side being stretched. Allow your head to return to neutral before releasing the wrist.

# Physioball Walk-up

### FEEL IT HERE: Legs, Hips, Core

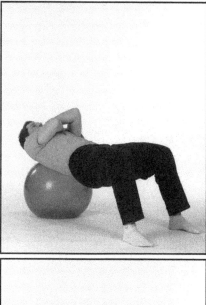
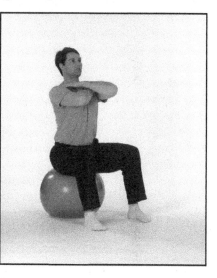
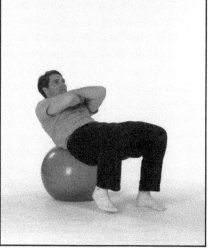

Position your hips on top of the physioball. Brace your core. Walk up the ball using your full foot. Keeping the feet wider adds stability if you feel off balance during the up or down phases.

# Lifting Movements with Band

### FEEL IT HERE: Core, Hips

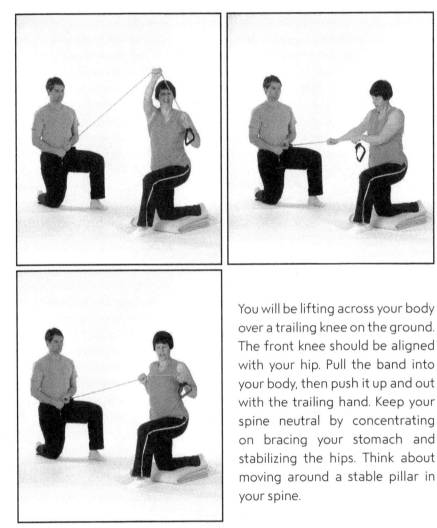

You will be lifting across your body over a trailing knee on the ground. The front knee should be aligned with your hip. Pull the band into your body, then push it up and out with the trailing hand. Keep your spine neutral by concentrating on bracing your stomach and stabilizing the hips. Think about moving around a stable pillar in your spine.

# CHAPTER 7

# Exercise Programs and Progressions

## PROGRAMMING FOR PARKINSON'S DISEASE

The programs outlined in this book follow a systematic approach to progress you from potentially a low level of total work capacity to one that meets the needs of your activities of improved daily living and beyond.

The following are the most up-to-date exercise guidelines, intended as recommendations for individuals with Parkinson's disease:

|  | **LEARNING PROGRAMS: THE BASICS** | **TRANSITIONAL PROGRAMS: FOCUSED HACKS** | **GENERAL HEALTH PROGRAMS** | **REASSESSMENT** |
|---|---|---|---|---|
| **Cycle** | 4–6 weeks | 4 weeks Pick 2–3 based on Assessments (page 121) | 8–12 weeks | 4 months Repeat Assessments |
| **Frequency** | 3–4 days/week | 2 non-consecutive days per week of work on areas needing improvement identified in the Assessments. | Minimum of 3 days per week, preferably 4 or more days per week that are most effective. Evaluate the following day for fatigue. | |
| **Intensity** | RPE of 3–5 out of 10 RPE scale. | Perform 45 seconds; RPE of 6 out of 10 RPE scale. | Perform 60 seconds; RPE of 7 out of 10 RPE scale. | |
| **Time** | 30 minutes total work time; 2 sets of 12 reps or 30–40 seconds/set | 45 minutes total work time 3 sets of 15 reps | 45 minutes total work time 3 sets of 15 reps | |
| **Type** | Various forms may be used, including but primarily body weight and bands. | Various forms may be used, not limited to body weight, bands, dumbbells. | Various forms may be used, including but not limited to body weight, bands, dumbbells. | |

| | FREQUENCY | INTENSITY | TIME | TYPE |
|---|---|---|---|---|
| Aerobic | Minimum of 2–3 non-consecutive days per week days per week, preferably 3 or more days per week. | 40–80 percent of exercise capacity. RPE of 12–16 on a scale of 6–20. | Begin with 5–10 steady state movement; build up to 20–30 minutes. If too difficult, break up into 2–3 segments of 10 minutes. | Various forms may be used: rower, treadmill, bike, elliptical |

| PROGRAM VARIABLES | TRANSITION WEEK | LEVEL 1 | LEVEL 2 | LEVEL 3 |
|---|---|---|---|---|
| Duration | 5 days | 2–4 weeks | 5–10 weeks | 2–4 weeks |
| Sets per exercise | Baseline | 1–3 | ≥ 3 | ≥ 3 |
| Reps per set | Baseline | 12–15 | 10–12 | 6–12 |
| Rest between sets | Baseline | 30 seconds | 30–60 seconds | 30–90 seconds |

## AEROBIC EXERCISE

While we often classify this area of an exercise prescription as aerobic, a better term may be cardiovascular, as it encompasses all three systems of energy development. Since each of these systems play a critical role in how we perform on a daily basis, it only makes sense that an exercise program will incorporate all three.

## STRENGTH TRAINING

Resistance training is an important component to any fitness program. This becomes even more evident when cardiac recovery is the focus. Not only does resistance training provide a stimulus to the cardiovascular system, it also increases our economy of movement, meaning that we become more efficient with our normal daily tasks or ADLs. Think about this way: if we increase our levels of muscular fitness (i.e. strength and endurance), everything we do becomes easier and thereby places less stress of the heart.

## MULTI-JOINT MOVEMENTS

When designing a resistance training program, including compound, multi-joint movements that work the major muscle groups of the body is a must. This includes exercises like squats, lunges, step-ups, upper body pushing and pulling, just to name few. We also include some single joint, isolation exercises as deemed appropriate. This is not only a time-efficient way to train, but also places the most demand and stimulus on the body creating a better dose response per workout. These exercises are also considered more functional in nature and have a better carryover to everyday life.

We will employ many of the same principles seen in the previous section for what is traditionally called aerobic fitness. The program will be progressive, adding both volume and intensity over the course of several weeks. This will allow for sufficient time to adapt to the new training stimulus. Unlike cardiovascular training, the frequency will be much less, based on the fact that more recovery is needed between sessions to allow the muscles involved to repair and regenerate, thereby getting stronger. Too much volume or frequency in the beginning will not allow you to have sufficient recovery between sessions.

You'll also find a programmed progression from variable resistance equipment (as found in most health clubs and fitness centers) to body weight and free weight exercises, and finally to suspension style exercises performed on a TRX Suspension System or similar equipment. This progression model helps to continuously overload the muscular system and provide a new training stimulus as you progress through the program. As you become familiar with the exercises, you may begin to systematically swap out exercises for other, biomechanically similar ones.

# The Complete Parkinson's Healthy Movement Program

## PROGRAMS

### Introductory
- Complete Mobility, Physical Assessments and Activities of Daily Living
- Complete Learning Program, Focus Points, Transitional Program and General Health progressions

### Beginner's Parkinson's Program
Using the results of your Assessments, determine what areas to concentrate on.

**Select workouts based upon those areas needing improvement/personal preference:**

- Posture
    + Start Workout A OR Start Workout B
- Balance
    + Start Workout A OR Start Workout B
- Core
    + Start Workout A OR Start Workout B
- Upper Body Flexibility
    + Start Workout A OR Start Workout B
- Lower Body Flexibility
    + Start Workout A OR Start Workout B
- General Mobility
    + Start Workout A OR Start Workout B
- Upper Body Strength
    + Start Workout A OR Start Workout B
- Lower Body Strength
    + Start Workout A OR Start Workout B

## Transition Programs
- Upper Body Transition
    + Upper Body Transition Workout A OR Upper Body Transition Workout B
- Lower Body Transition
    + Lower Body Transition Workout A OR Lower Body Transition Workout B

## General Health Programs: Integrated Full Body Workouts
- Start Progression Workout A
    + Morning Workout
    + Afternoon Workout
- Start Progression Workout B
    + Morning Workout
    + Afternoon Workout
- Start Progression Workout C
    + Morning Workout
    + Afternoon Workout

**Parkinson's Partner Programs: Family/Caregiver/ Home Health Aid**

- **Start Progression Workout A**
  + Morning Workout
  + Afternoon Workout
- **Start Progression Workout B**
  + Morning Workout
  + Afternoon Workout
- **Start Progression Workout C**
  + Morning Workout
  + Afternoon Workout

# PROGRESSIONS

Warm-up/warm-down refers to the number of minutes that should be taken to warm-up your body before a set of exercises and the time to warm-down your body. For example, 4/44 means that you should take 4 minutes to warm-up and 4 minutes to warm-down.

Rest refers to the time taken between each set of exercises.

RPE refers to Rate of Perceived Exertion. See page 41 for details.

# ASSESSMENTS

Based upon the outcome of your assessments, recommendations are provided for focus points.

## MOBILITY ASSESSMENT

| COMPLETE (YES/NO) DISCOMFORT (YES/NO) NOTE DIFFICULTY |
| --- |
| Heel to Toe Rocks |
| Single Leg Balancing/Weight Shifting |
| Overhead Squat (Hands on Wall) |
| Over/Under Back Scratch |
| Multi-Directional Patterns<br>    Forward Walk<br>    Backward Walk<br>    Backward Walk |

| |
|---|
| Lateral Slide |
| Up/Down from Chair (with/without hands) |

## PHYSICAL FITNESS ASSESSMENT

| COMPLETE (YES/NO) DISCOMFORT (YES/NO) NOTE DIFFICULTY |
|---|
| Stair Walking |
| Push-ups |
| Flex-Arm Hang (Optional) |
| Wall Sit with Foam Roller |
| Sitting or Standing with Eyes Open and Closed (Double/Single Leg) |
| Supermans |
| Glute Bridge |
| Stationary Lunge |

## ACTIVITIES OF DAILY LIVING (ADL) ASSESSMENT

| COMPLETE (YES/NO) DISCOMFORT (YES/NO) NOTE DIFFICULTY |
|---|
| Eating |
| Bathing |
| Getting Dressed |
| Toileting |
| Transferring (Walking) |
| Continence/Pelvic Floor Control |

# Learning Program: The Basics

## FOCUS: LEARNING BASICS A

**Reps:** 12–15 • **Sets:** 1–2 • **Rate of Perceived Exertion:** 2–4/10
Establishes body awareness utilizing the most stable position with the largest base of support.

| EXERCISE | PAGE # | EQUIPMENT/NOTES |
|----------|--------|-----------------|
| Ribs Heavy | 97 | |
| Hip Hinging | 58 | |
| Spinal Whip | 59 | |
| All 4s | 94 | |
| Glute Bridge | 79 | |

## FOCUS: LEARNING BASICS B

**Reps:** 10–12 • **Sets:** 1–2 • **Rate of Perceived Exertion:** 5/10

Advancing from ground-based to standing movements, integrating major movement areas: shoulder girdle, hip girdle and ankle complex. Progressively decreases base of support.

| EXERCISE | PAGE # | EQUIPMENT/NOTES |
|----------|--------|-----------------|
| Shoulder Circles | 60 | Foam roller |
| All 4s | 94 | |
| Glute Bridge | 79 | |
| Physioball Walk-Up | 114 | Physioball |
| Stationary Lunge | 81 | |

# Focus Points

## FOCUS: POSTURE WORKOUT A
**Reps:** 10–12 • **Sets:** 2 • **Rate of Perceived Exertion:** 5/10

| EXERCISE | PAGE # | EQUIPMENT/NOTES |
| --- | --- | --- |
| Lateral Neck Stretch | 113 | |
| Shoulder Circles | 60 | Foam roller |
| Thoracic Flex | 61 | Foam roller |
| Ribcage Opener | 67 | |
| Alphabet Series: Y | 65 | |

## FOCUS: POSTURE WORKOUT B
**Reps:** 12–15 • **Sets:** 3 • **Rate of Perceived Exertion:** 6/10

| EXERCISE | PAGE # | EQUIPMENT/NOTES |
| --- | --- | --- |
| Cranial Release | 62 | |
| Chin Tuck | 84 | |
| Alphabet Series: W | 66 | |
| Band Pulls | 109 | Band |
| Alphabet Series: T | 64 | |

## FOCUS: BALANCE WORKOUT A
**Reps:** 10–12 • **Sets:** • **Rate of Perceived Exertion:** 5/10

| EXERCISE | PAGE # | EQUIPMENT/NOTES |
| --- | --- | --- |
| Ankle Pumps | 68 | |
| Scissor Stretch | 63 | |
| Foot Taps | 92 | |
| Weight Shifting | 78 | |

## FOCUS: BALANCE WORKOUT B

**Reps:** 12–15 • **Sets:** 3 • **Rate of Perceived Exertion:** 6/10

| EXERCISE | PAGE # | EQUIPMENT/NOTES |
| --- | --- | --- |
| Foot Taps | 92 | |
| Towel Pulls | 75 | Towel |
| Calf/Shin Raise (Double Leg or Single Leg) | 70 | |
| Stationary Lunge | 81 | |

## FOCUS: CORE WORKOUT A

**Reps:** 10–12 • **Sets:** • **Rate of Perceived Exertion:** 5/10

| EXERCISE | PAGE # | EQUIPMENT/NOTES |
| --- | --- | --- |
| Kegels | 88 | |
| Forward Plank | 66 | |
| Lateral Plank | 57 | |
| Supermans to Prone Extension | 96 | |

## FOCUS: CORE WORKOUT B

**Reps:** 12–15 • **Sets:** 3 • **Rate of Perceived Exertion:** 6/10

| EXERCISE | PAGE # | EQUIPMENT/NOTES |
| --- | --- | --- |
| Thoracic Flex | 61 | Foam roller |
| All 4s | 94 | |
| Deadbug | 95 | |
| Physioball Walk-Up | 113 | Physioball |

## FOCUS: FLEXIBILITY WORKOUT A

**Reps:** 10–12 • **Sets:** • **Rate of Perceived Exertion:** 5/10

| EXERCISE | PAGE # | EQUIPMENT/NOTES |
| --- | --- | --- |
| Sitting Hip Stretch | 99 | |
| Scissor Stretch | 63 | Foam roller |
| Abductor Stretch | 106 | Foam roller |
| Chest Stretch (Wide Arms) | 76 | No partner |
| Thoracic Flex | 61 | Stick |

## FOCUS: FLEXIBILITY WORKOUT B

**Reps:** 12–15 • **Sets:** 3 • **Rate of Perceived Exertion:** 6/10

| EXERCISE | PAGE # | EQUIPMENT/NOTES |
|---|---|---|
| Quad Roller | 90 | Foam roller |
| Hip Roller | 89 | Foam roller |
| Cobra | 85 | |
| Alphabet Series: T | 64 | |

## FOCUS: GENERAL MOBILITY WORKOUT

**Reps:** 6–10 • **Sets:** 3 • **Rate of Perceived Exertion:** 7/10

| EXERCISE | PAGE # | EQUIPMENT/NOTES |
|---|---|---|
| Glute Bridge | 79 | |
| Hip Hinging | 58 | |
| Physioball Walk-Up | 113 | |
| Alternating Side/ Lateral Lunge to Clock Lunge | 100 | |
| Push-Ups | 53 | |

## FOCUS: UPPER BODY STRENGTH WORKOUT A

**Reps:** 10–12 • **Sets:** 3 • **Rate of Perceived Exertion:** 5/10

| EXERCISE | PAGE # | EQUIPMENT/NOTES |
|---|---|---|
| Shoulder Circles | 60 | Foam roller |
| Push-ups | 53 | |
| Band Rows | 73 | Band |
| Band Presses (Alternating) | 74 | Band |

# FOCUS: UPPER BODY STRENGTH WORKOUT B

**Reps:** 6–10 • **Sets:** 3–4 • **Rate of Perceived Exertion:** 7/10

| EXERCISE | PAGE # | EQUIPMENT/NOTES |
|---|---|---|
| Spinal Whip | 59 | |
| Band Pull-Aparts | 72 | |
| Lifting Movements with Band | 114 | Band |
| Dumbbell Row (Two Arms) | 56 | Dumbbells |
| Deadlift (Double Leg or Single leg) | 55 | Dumbell(s) |

# FOCUS: LOWER BODY STRENGTH WORKOUT A

**Reps:** 6–12 • **Sets:** 3–4 • **Rate of Perceived Exertion:** 7/10

| EXERCISE | PAGE # | EQUIPMENT/NOTES |
|---|---|---|
| Windshield Washer | 108 | |
| Glute Bridge | 79 | |
| Wall Sit with Foam Roller | 54 | Foam roller |
| Hip Lifters | 111 | |
| Single Leg Deadlift | 56 | Body weight |

# FOCUS: LOWER BODY STRENGTH WORKOUT B

**Reps:** 6–12 • **Sets:** 3–4 • **Rate of Perceived Exertion:** 7/10

| EXERCISE | PAGE # | EQUIPMENT/NOTES |
|---|---|---|
| Clock Lunge | 100 | |
| Push-ups | 53 | |
| Physioball Walk-Up | 113 | Physioball, dumbbell |
| Deadlift (Double Leg or Single Leg) | 56 | Dumbbell (optional) |
| Calf/Shin Raise (Double Leg or Single Leg) | 70 | |

# Transitional Workouts

## TRANSITIONAL WORKOUT A

**Reps:** 12 • **Sets:** 2 • **Rat of Perceived Exertion:** 5/10

| EXERCISE | PAGE # | EQUIPMENT/NOTES |
|---|---|---|
| All 4s | 94 | |
| Push-ups | 53 | |
| Lifting Movements with Band | 114 | Band |
| Physioball Walk-Up | 113 | |
| Clock Lunge | 100 | |

## TRANSITIONAL WORKOUT B

**Reps:** 10 • **Sets:** 3 • **Rate of Perceived Exertion:** 6/10

| EXERCISE | PAGE # | EQUIPMENT/NOTES |
|---|---|---|
| Band Presses (Alternating) | 74 | Band |
| Band Rows | 73 | Band |
| Band Pull-Aparts | 72 | Band |
| Stationary Lunge | 81 | Transition to Walking Lunge |

## TRANSITIONAL WORKOUT C

**Reps:** 15 • **Sets:** 3 • **Rate of Perceived Exertion:** 6/10

| EXERCISE | PAGE # | EQUIPMENT/NOTES |
|---|---|---|
| Dumbbell Row | 80 | Use band if preferred |
| Alternating Dumbbell Row (Double Arm) to Shoulder Press | 55 | Dumbbell |
| Push-ups | 53 | |
| Dumbbell Squat with Reach Across | 103 | Dumbbell |
| Forward Plank | 86 | |

## FOCUS: MULTITASKING INTEGRATED WORKOUT A
**Reps:** 12 • **Sets:** 3 • **Rate of Perceived Exertion:** 7/10

| EXERCISE | PAGE # | EQUIPMENT/NOTES |
|---|---|---|
| Quad Roller | 90 | Foam roller |
| Thoracic Flex | 61 | |
| Multiplanar Lunge Complex: Forward, Reverse, and Lateral | – | |
| Dumbbell Squat | 103 | Dumbbell(s) |
| Deadlift (Double leg or Single Leg | 56 | |
| Dumbbell Rows | 80 | Dumbbell(s) |
| Lifting Movements with Band | 114 | Band |

## FOCUS: MULTITASKING INTEGRATED WORKOUT B
**Reps:** 15 • **Sets:** 4 • **Rate of Perceived Exertion:** 8/10

| EXERCISE | PAGE # | EQUIPMENT/NOTES |
|---|---|---|
| Shoulder Circles | 60 | Foam roller |
| Hip Roller | 89 | Foam roller |
| Spinal Whip | 59 | |
| Push-ups | 53 | |
| Lateral Plank | 57 | |
| Walking Lunges | – | |
| Physioball Walk-Up with Curl | 113 | Physioball |

## FOCUS: MULTITASKING INTEGRATED WORKOUT C
**Reps:** 15 • **Sets:** 4 • **Rate of Perceived Exertion:** 8/10

| EXERCISE | PAGE # | EQUIPMENT/NOTES |
|---|---|---|
| All 4s | 94 | |
| Scissor Stretch | 63 | Foam roller |
| Deadlift (Double leg or Single Leg | 56 | |

| | | |
|---|---|---|
| Dumbbell Row (Double Arm) | 55 | Dumbbell(s) |
| Draw the Sword | 82 | Band |
| Curling and Pressing Combo | 110 | Dumbbell(s) |
| Band Pulls with One Knee Up | 107 | |

# Partner Programs: Family/ Caregiver/Home Health Aide

## PARTNER PROGRAM A
### Reps: 6–12 • Sets: 3–4 • Rate of Perceived Exertion: 7/10

| EXERCISE | PAGE # | EQUIPMENT/NOTES |
|---|---|---|
| Double Arm Chest Press | 102 | Dumbbell(s), partner |
| Single Arm Chest Press | 101 | Dumbbell(s), partner |
| Weight Shifting | 78 | Partner |
| Chest Stretch | 76 | Partner |

## PARTNER PROGRAM B
### Reps: 6–12 • Sets: 3–4 • Rate of Perceived Exertion: 7/10

| EXERCISE | PAGE # | EQUIPMENT/NOTES |
|---|---|---|
| Assisted Rotational Chair Stretch | 69 | Chair, partner |
| Partner Stability Pushes: Sitting and Standing | 77 | Partner |
| Back to Back Butterfly Stretch | 83 | Partner |
| Standing Double Arm Chest Press | 102 | Dumbbell(s) |
| Single Arm Chest Press | 101 | Dumbbell(s) |

# APPENDIX A:
## COMMONLY USED EXERCISE & HEALTH TERMINOLOGY

The following terms are often referenced in the health and exercise fields. We've included these commonly used terms as a point of reference.

**Acute Care:** Secondary health care in which a patient receives active short-term treatment for injury or illness, or during recovery from surgery.

**Blood Pressure:** Blood pressure can be broken down into two types: systolic and diastolic. Systolic is the pressure created when the heart exerts force, and diastolic is the pressure created upon the return of blood to the heart. Normal blood pressure is defined as 120/80, with the systolic figure on top, and diastolic figure on the bottom.

**Body Mass Index:** Also called BMI; a measurement of height and weight.

**Bradykinesia:** Slowness in initiating and executing movement.

**Bradyphrenia:** Slowness of thought process.

**Dyskinesia:** Involuntary movements (nodding, jerking, twisting), often resulting from medium to long-term use of certain medications.

**Fatigue:** A feeling of weariness and lethargy that persists over a long period of time and is not alleviated simply by rest.

**Orthostatic Hypotension:** A form of low blood pressure that occurs when standing up from sitting/lying down, which can make you feel dizzy and lightheaded.

**Outpatient Care:** Medical care provided on an outpatient basis, including diagnosis, observation, consultation, treatment, intervention, and rehabilitation services.

**Pulse Rate:** The number of heart beats per minute; the average resting rate for an adult is 60-80 BPM (beats per minute).

**Resting Heart Rate:** The number of times the heart beats per minute while resting; can be used as an indicator of physical fitness.

**Resting Tremor.** A tremor which occurs when the affected limb or body part is at rest. Can be exacerbated with stress.

**Restless Legs Syndrome:** An unrelated sensory disorder which commonly occurs in Parkinson's, characterized by the urge to move the legs during sleep or awake, at rest.

**Rigidity:** Muscle rigidity is felt on passive movement and may present as 'cogwheel' (when tremor is present) or 'lead-pipe' (in the absence of tremor).

**Sub-Acute:** A medical condition that falls between sudden onset (acute) and a condition with an indefinite duration (chronic).

**Syncope:** Partial or complete loss of consciousness caused by a sudden drop in blood pressure.

**Target Heart Rate Zone:** Also known as working rate; a personalized pulse rate to be maintained during exercise to reach optimal cardiovascular function; usually 60–85% of the maximum heart rate.

**Tremor:** An involuntary rhythmic movement which usually occurs when the affected body part is not in use (at rest). It may affect any part of the body but predominantly occurs in the upper or lower limbs or jaw and is initially seen on one side of the body. Internal tremors may be felt without being visible. Not all cases of Parkinson's will experience tremors.

# APPENDIX B:
# GLOSSARY OF EXERCISE TERMINOLOGY

**Aerobic:** Exercise that improves the efficiency of the cardiovascular system in obtaining oxygen from breathing.

**Anaerobic:** Short duration, high intensity exercise that is not intended to improve the cardiovascular system's ability to obtain oxygen from breathing.

**Closed Chain Exercise:** Exercises performed in which the hand or foot is in a fixed position and does not move.

**Compound Movement:** Exercises that engage multiple joints to train entire muscle groups.

**Load:** The amount of weight one lifts in relation to repetitions.

**Open Chain Exercise:** Exercises performed in which the hand or foot is free to move.

**Rate of Perceived Exertion (RPE):** A scale used to measure the perceived intensity of an exercise.

**Rate of Recovery:** The decrease in the heart rate from peak exercise until one minute after exercise ends.

**Repetition (Rep):** One complete motion of an exercise.

**Set:** A group of consecutive repetitions.

**Talk-test:** A test used to measure the intensity of an exercise; during moderate intensity you can talk, and during vigorous intensity you should not be able to say more than a few words without needing to take a breath.

**Volume:** The amount of work one does while exercising, such as the number of reps performed in one session.

**Work Rest Ration (W/R):** The amount of work (exercise) done in a session compared to the amount of rest.

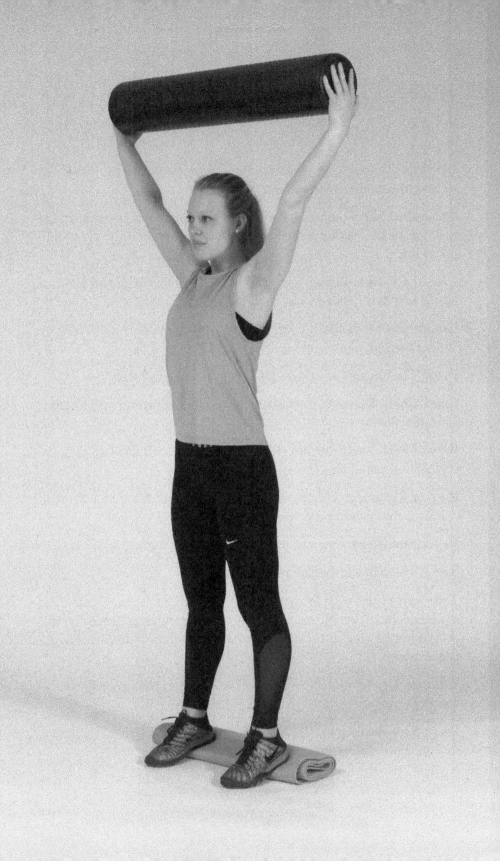

# RESOURCES

**National Organizations**
  **Parkinson's Disease Foundation**
    Website: http://www.parkinson.org/
    Toll Free Phone: 1-800-4PD-INFO (473-4636)

  **American Parkinson's Disease Association**
    Website: https://www.apdaparkinson.org/
    Toll Free Phone: 1-800-223-2732

  **Michael J. Fox Foundation for Parkinson's Research**
    Website: https://www.michaeljfox.org/
    Toll Free Phone: 1-800-708-7644

  **Davis Phinney Foundation for Parkinson's**
    Website: https://www.davisphinneyfoundation.org/
    Phone: 1-866-358-0285

**Additional Reading**
    National Parkinson's Foundation
    National Institute of Health: Parkinson's Disease
    National Institute of Neurological Disorders and Stroke
    National Institute on Aging
    American Parkinson Disease Association
    The Michael J. Fox Foundation for Parkinson's Research
    Bachman Strauss Dystonia & Parkinson Foundation
    Davis Phinney Foundation for Parkinson's
    Mayo Clinic: Parkinson's Disease Overview
    Morris K. Udall Parkinson's Disease Research Center for Excellence
    (Johns Hopkins University)

**Social Groups**
  **Healthline**
    https://www.healthline.com/health/parkinsons/best-blogs-of-the-year#2

### Everything about Parkinson's Disease

This group is for all people afflicted with Parkinson's, their caregivers and family. Members can feel free to share personal experiences about PD, the latest scientific news, articles, disease management tips and more.

### Caregivers of Parkinson's Disease Support Group

This group is strictly for caregivers of Parkinson's disease patients and their loved ones.

# ABOUT THE AUTHOR

**William Smith, MS, NSCA-CSCS, MEPD,** currently works for a nationally recognized healthcare system in the New York metropolitan area providing health and wellness services to the community. His interest is in special populations and how healthcare providers and fitness professionals can work more closely together.

Will completed his B.S. in exercise science followed by an MS at St. John's University where he was the Assistant Director of Strength and Conditioning. Will has been featured on NBC, Canyon Ranch, World Spinning Conference and in Homecare Magazine.

## ALSO IN THIS SERIES